"WHY DID MY BABY DIE?"

"WHY DID MY BABY DIE?"

Abraham B. Bergman, M.D.
and
Judith Choate

The Third Press
Joseph Okpaku Publishing Company, Inc.
444 Central Park West, New York, N.Y. 10025

Library of Congress Catalog Card Number: 73-92794
ISBN 0-89388-146-5

First printing 1975

Designed by Bennie Arrington

CONTENTS

PREFACE

"Every night several million American mothers feed their babies, put them in their cribs, and say good night. The next morning they return, greet their children and begin another day of care. Yet every morning, anywhere from 30 to 60 mothers return to find their babies lying dead in their cribs—victims of a mysterious and frightening disease that takes the lives of at least 10,000 infants each year.

Some people know this disease by the name of 'crib death' or 'cot death.' Others call it 'Sudden Infant Death Syndrome.' By any name, it is an elusive disease which strikes not only the child, but his whole family. Sometimes the victim's parents and brothers and sisters never recover from the shock, guilt and self-incrimination that follow."

> Senator Walter F. Mondale
> January 25, 1972
> United States Senate Subcommittee
> on Children and Youth Hearing on
> the Sudden Infant Death Syndrome

Five years ago this book couldn't have been written. The Sudden Infant Death Syndrome (SIDS) was, at that time, still an unrecognized entity known only to a few research physicians, medical examiners, coroners and the unfortunate families who had lost babies. Through consumer action plans organized by parent groups, remarkable changes have occurred. More research has been done in the past five years than had been done in the previous five hundred. More communities are offering adequate services to the stricken families. More physicians recognize that although finding a cause and cure is a top priority requiring vast amounts of time and money, much can be done to support the family which requires no money and little time. Legislative action, on both the federal and state levels, continues to lighten the burden of the lay group. In total, families of the future can have some assurance that although the key to the prevention of the syndrome may still be years away, should they lose a child to the syndrome, they will be treated with understanding, dignity and compassion.

In 1965, the authors of this book were deeply affected by the still little-known disease: one by choice and one by fate.

ABRAHAM BERGMAN

"I was a typical young practitioner of 'academic medicine.' School, at long last, was over and I had just 'settled down.' For physicians, this means completion of college, medical school, internship, residency, service time and for those headed for faculty positions, fellowship training. Having been away from my hometown, Seattle, for 13 years engaged in these pursuits, I was eager to return. A former teacher of mine in medical school at Cleveland, Dr. Ralph Wedgwood, had become the chairman of the Pediatrics Department at the University of Washington, and when he offered me a position on his faculty, I enthusiastically accepted.

My base of operations was the Children's Orthopedic Hospital and Medical Center, where I was responsible for the operation of the Outpatient Department. Most medical school faculty members also engage in research; my specialty was research in 'medical care' or, more specifically, how to improve health services by more creative utilization of manpower.

Another new arrival at the Children's Hospital and the

medical school was Dr. J. Bruce Beckwith, who had come
from Los Angeles. With a unique blend of brilliance and
charm, this young pathologist attracted a devoted following.
His research interest was 'crib death.' The sum and substance of my education on the subject throughout medical
school and pediatric training was limited to a solitary lecture
delivered to my medical school fraternity by a Cleveland
pathologist, Dr. Lester Adelson.

Beckwith wanted to continue his pathology study on crib
death, which he had began in Los Angeles, and wanted a
pediatrician to collaborate with him to obtain interviews
from families in their homes. I volunteered. It didn't take
longer than the first home interview to recognize that I had
not embarked on an ordinary research project. As soon as
I had finished asking my questions, I witnessed what was to
become a repetitive scene: stunned parents asking, 'Why did
my baby die?' Behind the spoken question lay the unspoken
one: 'Was I responsible for my baby's death?' We had
stumbled upon another research project that was wholly
unanticipated; what happens to families who suffer the
sudden and unexpected loss of a loved baby.

My component of the Seattle research project completed,
and other interests beckoning, I had thought that my appearance at the Chicago Parent Medical Conference in 1971
would mark the end of my active involvement with SIDS.
I had not reckoned on the poignant power of bewildered
parents from all across the country seeking help. A young
woman stopped me in the lobby of the hotel with tears in
her eyes and said, 'Can you tell me why my baby died?' We
sat down and it turned out that she was the wife of a young
Chicago surgeon. She pulled a crumpled piece of paper out
of her purse—the death certificate—and handed it to me.
On it were the words, 'tracheobronchitis staph aureus.' The
story she told was the classic one for SIDS. I told her, 'It

appears that your baby died of Sudden Infant Death Syndrome.' 'Why didn't anybody tell me, and why did I have to have a coroner's inquest?' she burst out. I said, 'What does your husband say?' She turned her face away and said, 'He can't talk about it.' My consciousness was stabbed. 'If such things happen to physicians' families, how on earth must other families in the United States, who lose children to crib death be treated,' I thought.

The more families I met, the more my grim suspicions were confirmed. The management of Sudden Infant Death Syndrome in the United States was a national disgrace and something had to be done. I also met Judith Choate and I was 'hooked' into the national campaign to humanize the handling of SIDS."

JUDITH CHOATE

"I was a young, rather inexperienced New York housewife with little interest in medicine except as it insured the well-being of my two sons, Michael, 3 years, and Robert, 5 months. On a March morning, my life changed with a sharp jolt and a part of medicine became an all-consuming interest. My five-month-old son was discovered lifeless in his crib. No warning sickness, no struggle, no cry. Another tiny victim of crib death.

Like all cases of sudden, unexpected and unattended deaths in our city, Robbie was a Medical Examiner's case. His body was left in the apartment, in a closed bedroom, with a policeman in attendance until mid-afternoon when a medical investigator (from the Medical Examiner's office) observed the body and interviewed us. Questions such as 'How many times did you hit the baby?', 'Did your other child choke or in any way abuse the baby?' provoked a commitment to protect every SIDS family from the agony of feeling responsible for their child's death. I can remember wondering, as they took the baby to the morgue, what happens to families who don't speak English, who have never heard of crib death, who don't have private medical care. I suppose it was, in part, easier to think about abstracts than to face my own terror. I spent a manic day trying to track down a foundation concerned with crib deaths. I had read about it, I knew it was in Connecticut. I knew it was a child's name and I knew I had to help. I called every medical school, library and hospital in New York with no results. No one knew what I was talking about. I finally started calling the major women's magazines. At the moment they took the baby's body from the apartment, I was given the name of the Mark Addison Roe Foundation by the editor of a national publication.

I had enough knowledge about crib death to know that the foundation could not tell me why Robbie died, but that was not my need. I just wanted to help in any way I could; thus, one week later when I began to correspond with other parents across the country, I did not know that my involvement would be long-term nor did I suspect the horror stories I would come to know well. I guess I have kept going with the thought that although I could never save a baby's life, I could help insure that someone would try. Also I could try to save families from the anguish and misery of holding themselves responsible for the death of their child."

At opposite coasts of the United States, the authors pursued their particular interests in the problem: one in a community where families were receiving the best possible treatment; the other involved with families throughout the United States, most of whom received no treatment at all.

Through the years, each had developed strong ideas on what could be done to lift the veil of ignorance and apathy surrounding the problem.

In 1971, they met, for the first time, when both were speakers at the First National Parent-Medical Conference on Sudden Infant Death Syndrome. Although they had been separated by thousands of miles and were involved in quite different aspects, both spoke about the same thing—the humanization of the handling of the Sudden Infant Death Syndrome. Out of this evolved a partnership that would lead a national volunteer effort to eradicate the psychological toll of the Sudden Infant Death Syndrome, and to foster research which would eventually end the problem entirely. The effort is beginning to show effect.

II

WHY DID MY BABY DIE?

"What did I do? Healthy babies don't just die. Please help me understand how I killed my little girl."

SIDS Parent—1972

Sudden Infant Death Syndrome is a double crisis: a human one with far-reaching psychological effects, as well as a biomedical one with no preventive measures. We will begin with the human aspect. The following letters have been chosen from among those received during the past ten years by the National Foundation for Sudden Infant Death, Inc.

Some are from parents who lost their babies many years ago and know nothing of crib death. Some are from parents who have had immediate contact with someone who knew something about the disease. The only common bond they have is a sense of responsibility for the death.

The guilt feelings are a natural reaction to an event that defies rational explanation. However, when the community around them also points an accusing finger, the feelings of self-incrimination are intensified.

Virtually every parent has a theory to explain the child's death and a great many feel their loss could have been prevented. Allergy to milk, caught in the crib covers, a cold that should have been treated in a hospital, and so on, *ad infinitum*. Without adequate and immediate explanation by

a qualified health professional, these theories tend to dom-
inate the event and further intensify the guilt.

"We lost our little boy and I have just read a column about
what maybe killed him. He didn't have an autopsy but
everything I have read or heard about crib death points to
that as the cause of his going away. He was 7 months old
and had a little cold but his last night on earth he seemed
perfectly healthy and happy. I found him the next morning
dead.

It is so hard to write about it now as I feel absolutely
horrified. I have another little boy and a loving husband
and I know that somehow I must go on. I feel that reading
this column must be God's answer to me. I feel so guilty
and heartbroken and responsible for all this. He was so
perfect. Can you please help our family to go on and maybe
you can show me the way to do this? I am sending you a
picture of the baby so you can see how sweet he was. This
terrible thing of crib death must be stopped. How do
mothers go on? I want more children but then I ask myself
if my mistakes harmed the baby; and how will I ever really
know what mistakes I made so I won't do it again. Please
help me!"

"I read an article on infant deaths and would like more
information. I had a 3-month-old-baby boy die about 39
years ago and at that time we had two doctors examine him
and both only said 'It is just one of those things.' They did
say that they probably couldn't have saved him. I have
always wanted more information.

He was a twin and my other son has always been very
healthy. The one who died had been healthy also but he
had the flu a week prior to his death. Do you think he could
have had pneumonia and I did not know it? I was so young
and inexperienced.

When the other baby got sick afterwards I went to a different doctor. I had lost faith in the doctor who could not give me any comfort at all about my baby who died so suddenly. I have never forgotten this and although I am a great-grandmother now I still would like to know why my baby died.

Thank you."

"I am 18 years old, my husband is 21. We were married October 12, 1968. June 19, 1969 we had a baby girl. She would have been three months old September 19, 1969— the day she died.

We had left her with my mother-in-law for 3 days. We went to pick her up the evening of September 18, 1969. My mother-in-law informed me she thought the baby was catching a cold. She said she had a runny nose.

She was in a playful mood when we arrived home. My husband wanted me to let her stay up later and play. However, I had her on a schedule. She was to go to bed at 9:00 p.m.; she usually woke up at about 7:00 a.m. Then after she had her bath and ate she usually went back to sleep for an hour or two.

I put Vicks on her back, chest and throat—then I put a heating pad under her sheet and turned it on to medium.

I worked from the time she was 2 weeks old until she was about 2½ months. (My husband was in jail at this time, that's why we left her at my mother-in-law's—because he just got out and we wanted to be alone—so we could go places and have fun.)

So, she was used to being with her grandmother and uncles. Naturally she was spoiled and didn't like to go to bed. So she cried until about 10 or 10:30. At 11:00 just before we went to bed my husband went in to check on her. She was asleep on her stomach (she wouldn't sleep on her back). He asked me to come in the bedroom and showed me that she was covered with perspiration, her clothes were soaked. I presumed the heating pad was on too high although it didn't feel too warm when I touched it. I turned it on low. We had just moved to the apartment and didn't have the heat turned on yet so I didn't want to turn the heating pad all the way off.

At about 2:30 or 3:00 I woke up. The baby was screaming—not just crying but screaming. I thought that she just had a bad dream. I went to her room and tried to give her a bottle, but she wouldn't take it. She just kept on screaming. I went back to bed and she shut up in about 15 or 20 minutes—but all this time she was screaming.

At 6:00 we got up because I was going to take my husband to look for a job. I went in to get her to give her a bath. I picked her up and she was stiff—I dropped her back down. Her little fists were purple and they were gripping the sheet. There was white foam in her mouth.

The coroner said she had been dead probably 3 or 4 hours. I guess she stopped crying when she died. They said it was crib death but never did tell me anything more than that. I think she suffocated from the heat of the heating pad. My husband and mother-in-law both told me that it wasn't because of the heating pad and told me to call the autopsy man a few days later when I was off tranquilizers. He again told me it was crib death. But no one ever told me what that meant.

We now have a 7-month-old baby. When he was 5 months old he was put in the hospital for 3 days for what doctors thought was bronchitis. They found he was only sick from allergy to a drug another doctor had prescribed for his cold while my baby's doctor was away.

The first day he went to the hospital my husband and

I got into an argument. He said I never took care of the baby and that it was my fault he was in the hospital.

We were living with my mother-in-law then, too (neither her nor my father-in-law could drive so I had to take each of them back and forth to work every day plus I had to do all the housework). So, about all I could do with the baby was give him a bath and my husband took care of him the rest of the time.

Also when he said it was my fault that the baby was in the hospital, he said "At least I never killed our little girl." He had never said that to me before and didn't mean to say it then, it just slipped out. But that proved to me that he does think I killed her. Since then, I wonder all the time if it was my fault and if I really did kill her with the heating pad. Maybe my mother-in-law and the autopsy guy know I killed her with the heating pad and are hiding it from me. I don't know why, but I feel that they are lying to me. I am afraid to ask my husband.

(THIS LETTER GOES ON FOR THREE MORE PAGES PLEADING FOR ANSWERS TO QUESTIONS RELATED TO SLEEP, EATING HABITS, ETC. BUT IS MAINLY REPETITIVE.)

Well, there are probably more questions I could ask, but I mainly want to know if you think I killed my baby or did she really die from crib death? And what is crib death? Please help me as soon as possible. I don't want to kill my new baby."

"It was six days before Christmas when our world seemed to fall in on us. We had put our son to bed the night before when we went in to get him in the morning he was gone. He cried out about 6:30 but he didn't seem mad and after a minute he quit crying. I laid in bed until about 7:00. I put his bottle on and went to peek at him. He was snuggled up under the covers, face down. His little hand was sticking out and I knew something was wrong before I uncovered him.

We have relived the tragedy over and over again in our minds. What if we had gone to him at 6:30 that morning, would it have made a difference. There should have been some warning or something to be alerted for. He was a good eater and was gaining weight. At his check-up he was fine and healthy. So how could he be gone?

The reason for this letter is we would like to be on your mailing list. Plus, maybe you could tell us how a healthy baby could die.

We are also expecting a new baby and we need some reassurance. We are so scared but happy. Do other parents have fears as a new baby comes? What about clothes and furniture of the lost baby? Should they be used again? Are there any virus or germs on them?

Thank you for helping us."

"Our first grandson was born in November. He was a perfect baby in every way. His father, our son, is a doctor in the Service. Our daughter-in-law is very efficient and a good mother and the baby was so wanted.

They put him to bed on a December evening and one half hour later when they went in to check him, he was dead. He was breastfed and seemed to be healthy. Not even a sniffle or sign of a cold. Our son rushed him to the hospital but to no avail. He was 6 weeks and 1 day old.

Our son and his wife are very broken up over this even though he is a doctor. This was their first child and we are all just crushed. If he had been ill or if his birth wasn't accepted (in other words, if this baby wasn't wanted) perhaps it would be easier to bear but that is just not the case. They want to have other children but we are all so terribly concerned. Could there be anything in our family or did my children miss something?

We would appreciate whatever help you can give us."

"On September 6, my huband and I were blessed with a baby boy. On November 7, he died. I checked on him early in the morning. He had died during his sleep. We rushed him to the hospital and the nurses took him away. At that time, I was very emotional. My parents came and after I had received the news they took me home. I felt that I had not given the baby the best care. I have blamed myself for a long time and still feel guilty for perhaps not giving our son the attention I should have. From that day on, I was very sheltered by my husband. He took full control of all arrangements. We never speak of our son. I have never fully understood his death. Since then we have not had another child. I would like to have your booklet and I would also like to know who I ask for a full report on the cause of his death. An autopsy was not performed but I was never told the exact cause of his death. Thank you for your help."

"I had a baby die of crib death three years ago. We didn't have an autopsy and we were told that she died of a virus in the lungs. We never did get any certificate or anything. The doctor who was taking care of the baby didn't tell us anything either. He just said we should have other children and forget about the baby who died.

I can't forget about the baby. She was my only daughter and I loved her so much. My mother thinks that I maybe shouldn't have put new blankets in the crib but I wanted her to have everything new and pink so I did. Do you think that the blanket killed her? I know that I did something wrong because babies don't just die like that. She was blond and blue-eyed and so pretty and was never sick at all and

she was only 2 months old. My husband won't talk about it
—he thinks it is something in our genes that killed her.
Why did she die and our sons live, then? What did I do
wrong? Please help me."

"In reading a column in our local newspaper we heard of
other bereaved parents of a victim of crib death and the
subsequent inhuman investigation amounting to almost a
"third degree." Having spent years in a hospital, I am aware
of brutality to infants but how can one look at a dead infant
with grief stricken parents in a state of shock and be unaware of true grief?

Our daughter lost her only baby at the age of 7 months
from crib death and was subjected to such an investigation
by the D.A. and the sheriff, also at the hospital. She was in
such a state of shock herself that she had to be tranquilized
and hospitalized. She has never nor will she ever forget the
torture while standing over her dead boy that both she and
her husband adored.

I wish we could help more in devising a better system of
dealing with these families. No one should have to go
through what my daughter experienced.

Thank you for all you are doing."

"My husband and I thank you so much for the literature
you sent about SIDS. We are parents who did not order an
autopsy (regrettably now) but who, after having read the
material, are more convinced than ever that we lost our
daughter of five months to the Sudden Infant Death Syndrome. Like many other parents we thought when we found
her that somehow she had suffocated and the physician who
examined her and tried in vain to revive her accepted this
assumption also. This was even recorded on her death certificate. It was later that the questions began, not only from

ourselves, but from friends and relatives. How could she have smothered when there were no blankets or pillows anywhere near her? And how could the doctor have accepted such an explanation and not suggest we have an autopsy?

I'm sure I don't have to tell you the agonizing weeks we suffered, especially my parents who still wonder if the home-made crib (made for her first visit to her grandparents) had something to do with the baby's death. While I am quite ignorant about autopsies, if I thought one could still be performed after an exhumation, I would have it now to convince my parents that our little baby could not have suffocated. I ask you, are they ever performed under such circumstances or as I fear would it be way too late to obtain significant results?

Thank heavens for the work you are doing. Thank you for being there for all parents who need you. I feel that I can now get through another day."

"I need your help. My 2-month-old daughter has died and I love her very much. It was our first child. She was born on January 31—she died April 1.

My baby—I carried her for nine months. She weighed 8 pounds 2½ ounces, she never lost any weight she gained. When she died she weighed 14 pounds and was very happy. She ate good, slept good.

Our family got the flu. I was wondering if my baby could of gotten the flu without anyone knowing about it. The only thing that happened was that I did not realize 'til she died that for three days before she died she slept two days and I had to wake her up to feed her. Then the next day she was all right. That night I gave her supper then I put her to bed. She seemed restless but everybody told me that lots of babies do cry all night and are all right. Well, I picked her up and rocked her to sleep. She was breathing okay. She didn't act like she had a cold or anything. The next morning she was dead.

Now I am a nervous wreck. I don't care if I live or not. The man that checks dead people said there was no sense in doing anything to her because they won't find anything. I am heartbroken.

What I want to know is do you have any idea what could have been wrong with her? They told me it might be crib death—what is that—I don't believe that my baby or any baby could die from nothing.

We want to have more children but I am scared to become pregnant because I am afraid it will happen again. I just can't take it anymore. I am on nerve pills. I keep hearing her crying. I don't feel like seeing my friends because when I do I don't know what to say to them. I need your help. I am going to end up in a mental hospital if I don't get some help from someone soon. I am so lonely."

"I am very interested in helping your organization with public awareness on the different aspects of Sudden Infant Death.

I have followed the Senate investigations through the news media. But I want to do something about it! Be an active participator. Possibly my circumstances will be different.

My first son (my only son) was born in 1966. He weighed 7 lbs. 8 oz., was 21″ long and was just fine. A week later, my neighbor gave birth to a girl, it was a joke of how they would probably be sweethearts. Both babies prospered. Three months later, my girl friend's baby was found dead in her crib. A victim of crib death. I was so stunned I couldn't think of words to comfort the parents, who were my friends.

At home, no one talked much about the "lost baby" but rather of the parents.

On Sunday, a week later, we all slept late. I got breakfast ready and went upstairs to get the children. My daughter, age 15 months, was wide awake in her crib; I glanced over at my son's crib and he was still sleeping. I brought my daughter downstairs and put her into her high chair, set her breakfast in front of her and went to get my husband up. He sat down at the kitchen table, I poured him coffee and went upstairs to bring my son down. I looked at him and he seemed so peaceful. I began to pick him up and his hand was limp. I looked at his face—one side was white, the other was blue. I screamed for my husband and we shook him and nothing! I ran downstairs and called the police. (At the time, we lived in a small town of 1500 people.) I ran outside to get a neighbor to care for my daughter, as the police car pulled in.

The policeman didn't ask me any questions. He picked up my son, and laid him on the sofa and began to give him mouth-to-mouth resuscitation. The police chief then came in and asked us for our pediatrician's name and phone number. The doctor was in a town some 15 miles away and of course, no one could reach him. There were 3 doctors in our town but none of them would come to the house. The chief called for an ambulance with first-aid team. It took half an hour. As they pulled in with their oxygen, I had hope. The police chief asked us a few questions regarding the health of the baby and the circumstances regarding him and how I found him. I was terrified, I answered the questions, but I knew they would think I did something to him.

The oxygen brought color into his face and I felt sure he would live. The ambulance men were going to take him to the nearest hospital which is 18 miles away, as there would be a doctor there. Just as they carried him out to the ambulance, our family dentist, who lived 2 houses away came over with a bag to see if he could help. He was the only doctor willing to try, and he advised us to go to the hospital.

As we got to the emergency room door of the hospital, we could see the ambulance backing in. The available doctor wouldn't even allow my son into the hospital. He examined him quickly in the ambulance, said he was 'sorry' and said he had been dead quite awhile. I never saw my son again.

The police asked us a few more questions as to where we wanted the body taken, etc. and the rest was all routine.

Two weeks later, a baby at the other end of town died the same way and the three babies are all buried together.

I couldn't really thank the police for their help. They were wonderful. But the doctors involved, as well as the pathologist, and the medical examiner should have been brought before some board of inquiry as to why they wouldn't come to our house and why they kept questioning over and over again.

It took me five years to decide to have another baby; plus I left my husband. We kept blaming each other and it got worse. I remarried and had another baby girl. The first three or four months were hard. I couldn't bear to go into her room and check on her. I also had a pediatrician who would come to the house. I moved to a large city and I am 5 minutes from 2 hospitals.

Even though I've changed my entire life style, I still have the nightmares and the eerie feeling in my heart. If I only knew why. How could this happen? What causes this?

Please help me to get involved in this. Is there a group in my town formed of parents who have lost babies this way? What can be done?"

III

THE HISTORY OF SUDDEN INFANT DEATH SYNDROME

"And this woman's child died in the night because she overlaid it—and she rose at midnight
and took my son from beside me, while thine
hand maid slept and laid it on her bosom and laid
her dead child on my bosom."

I Kings 3:19,22

Crib death has been with us since antiquity, but disguised under a variety of names and surrounded by mystery and superstition. In fact, it was not until 1969 that the term "Sudden Infant Death Syndrome" began to be applied to what was finally recognized by scientists as a distinct disease entity.

In biblical times sudden infant deaths were attributed to "overlaying." At the time it was common practice to put small babies to sleep in the same bed with their parents, siblings or a nurse. It was a widely held belief that infants suffocated when an adult or older child rolled over on them during sleep. If the Bible had recorded the complete conversation of King Solomon and the two women who both claimed the surviving infant, perhaps his wisdom might have comforted parents through the ages. We only know that he suggested the infant be cut in half and that it was restored to its rightful mother when she offered to give up the claim rather than see the child harmed. We are not told

19

what happened to the mother whose child was "overlaid," but it is safe to assume that her life was not easy.

Prior to the 19th century, and indeed, well into our own, sudden deaths of infants were not viewed with any particular alarm. Smallpox, diptheria, scarlet fever, cholera, whooping cough, and other diseases took their toll of all ages; small children were merely considered particularly vulnerable. It was not until the middle of the 19th century that crib death even began to be considered as a separate medical problem.

In an 1893 edition of the *Edinburgh Medical Journal*, Dr. Charles Templeman, a Scottish physician, reported a study of 399 cases of sudden infant deaths over a ten year period in the city of Dundee, Scotland. As a police surgeon, Templeman, personally examined 258 of the children who died unexpectedly in that industrial city with a population of over 150,000. He ascribed the cause of death to suffocation and suggested these deaths tended to be confined to the lower classes, ". . . parents were of dissipated and dissolute habits, living amidst squalor and filth. . . ." He believed the principal causes of this sort of death were ". . . ignorance, and carelessness of mothers, drunkenness, overcrowding and illegitimacy." Templeman strongly believed these infant deaths could be prevented and that the responsibility should be placed on someone, with criminal charges being brought against the parents. He proposed a modification of a 13th century German law which prohibited adults and older children from sleeping in the same bed with children under the age of two.

Dr. Templeman performed postmortem examinations on a minority of the 258 infants. His findings, though, appear to be consistent with those of present day pathologists: ". . . fluid condition of the blood . . . small punctiform hemorrhages observed beneath the pleura and pericardium; larynx, trachea and bronchi were, as a rule, congested."

Unfortunately, the theories of Templeman persisted well into our own century despite a very large logical inconsistency. Were crib death due to suffocation, one would expect the tiniest and weakest of babies to be the most vulnerable. Such was (and is) not the case; babies in the first few weeks of life are generally spared, with the peak incidence of crib death occuring between the second and fourth month of age.

Another theory which was widely believed, and regrettably still convinces the uneducated, is that of aspiration of stomach contents, babies "choking on their milk." It is not hard to understand why this "aspiration theory" was so popular. After a person dies, from whatever cause, the muscles controlling the inner organs (sphincters) relax, including the sphincters of the digestive tract. If a person is lying down, any food present in the stomach flows back up into the mouth and into the breathing tubes of the lungs. Thus little babies who die commonly have milk curds distributed through their lungs. It is then understandable why an uninformed person may believe that milk in the lung was the cause of death.

With the appearance of medical journals sudden infant deaths are frequently mentioned. An 1842 *American Journal of Medical Science* article proposed the theory of the enlarged thymus as an explanation for these deaths, previously ascribed to suffocation. While the theory later fell into disrepute, it did serve to lay the blame on a medically diagnosable condition, thereby shifting the responsibility from the parents. It again became popular in the 1930's among the "modern" doctors, who used the impressive term "status thymicolymphaticus" to describe crib death. Again their observations were correct and the reasoning wrong.

The thymus gland, now known to be important in the development of the child's immune defense system, is at its largest during the first six months of life. It is a gland that overlies the heart and windpipe, contains much fat, and shrinks very rapidly during periods of severe illness or malnutrition. The vast majority of babies who died during the first year of life, were either malnourished or had severe illnesses. At autopsy, their thymus glands were small. In contrast, children dying suddenly and unexpectedly were found to have much larger thymus glands. Again it was believed that the "enlarged" thymus had somehow compressed the heart and lungs causing the death. Medicine in the 1930's did not see that it was the large thymus glands that were normal and the small ones that were abnormal. So sure were some doctors of this theory, that it became common practice for normal infants to be x-rayed to see if their glands were "enlarged." Infants with glands thought to be too large were given x-ray therapy to shrink the gland as a preventative measure against crib death. Sadly, the dangers of radiation were not appreciated at that time, and a goodly number of the youngsters who were given this treatment developed cancer of the thyroid in later years.

The major reason for the dearth of knowledge about crib death was simply the lack of organized research efforts devoted to the subject. Research is not easy. Contrary to popular image, rarely does it involve geniuses waiting for apples to fall on their heads. Flashes of inspiration are not enough. Research is an *organized* search for knowledge. Creativity is finding productive *methods* whereby problems can be studied. Too many "Walter Mittys" want to perform armchair research, and hope that lightning will strike. The public hears much about spectacular breakthroughs, and little about the years of painstaking background work leading up to them.

Also, talent and the problem had to be brought together. The people most capable of performing scientific work simply were unaware of the existence of the problem of crib death. Some of the great discoveries in medicine have come about because the curiosity of talented scientists were aroused by the problems they saw in hospitals. Crib death victims did not go to hospitals, or if they did, it was only to be pronounced dead in an emergency room and then transferred quickly to a local morgue. They were little seen, and even less heard by the group who could have helped most.

There were a few voices in the wilderness. While crib death was a problem remote from doctors and hospitals and medical schools, it was well known to the fellow working in the county morgue. The overworked and underpaid coroner and medical examiner offices must be credited with finally setting crib death research on the right path to solid answers.

It all began with a series of papers from the office of the Chief Medical Examiner in Queens, New York, between 1942 and 1953. Drs. Werne and Garrow presented strong evidence to suggest a natural and probably inflammatory mechanism as a cause of sudden infant death. They thoroughly discounted the "prevalent suffocation theories."

Dr. Clara Raven, working in the office of the Wayne County Medical Examiner in Detroit, also found inflammatory changes in the lungs and suggested the possibility that viruses were involved in the crib death process.

Then a notable paper appeared in the *Journal of Pediatrics* in 1945 written by Dr. Paul V. Wooley, a pediatrician at the University of Oregon who later moved to the Children's Hospital in Detroit. Wooley was skeptical of the prevailing suffocation theory and made a study that is probably impermissible today amidst the tide of controversy about "human experimentation." He attached a photoelectric cell to the ear lobes of several infants, a procedure which measures the amount of oxygen in the blood. He then tightly covered their faces with blankets while they were asleep. He found not only that the babies continued to sleep, but that the oxygen concentration in their blood remained perfectly normal even while they were breathing through bed clothes. Dr. Wooley proved conclusively that it is impossible for a normal child to smother in his bed clothes.

IV

CRIB DEATH RESEARCH
BECOMES RESPECTABLE

"It seems probable that at least in most instances
these deaths do represent a single disease entity.
The bulk of them are due to a single pathologic
mechanism. Progress towards the discovery of the
mechanism would seem to require at the outset
recognition of the scope of our present ignorance."

> Maria A. Valdes-Dapena
> The Scope of Our Ignorance
> *Pediatric Clinics of North America*
> August 1963

If the modern era of crib death research started in the
forties and fifties, it still remained outside the regular channel of scientific activity until the 1960's. The First International Conference on the Causes of Sudden Death in
Infants in Seattle in September of 1963 marks the point
when crib death research finally became respectable. With
a full dose of cynicism intended, it seems safe to surmise
that the subject might not have been discussed at a scientific meeting until the year 2063 had not a small band of
bereaved and militant parents stood up and demanded action.
Change was prompted by individuals, rather than by organizations. Mary and Fred Dore were two of those dedicated
individuals.

State Senator and Mrs. Dore live in Seattle, Washington.
They lost their fourth child, a three-month-old-daughter, to

crib death on September 8, 1961. Her case was like so many others. The baby had been fussy the night before and Mary had been up several times in the night tending to her. She was rushed to the County hospital and pronounced dead on arrival. An autopsy was performed and "acute pneumonitis" listed on the death certificate. The coroner spent some time explaining "acute pneumonitis" to the parents, telling them it was a catchall phrase to include the sudden and unexpected deaths of previously healthy infants. In the course of their conversation, the coroner told the Dores that he'd seen 30 to 50 such cases every year in the Seattle-King County area. Fred and Mary had heard vaguely of crib death before, but were shocked to learn of its prevalence in their own community. They worried about the term "pneumonia" on the death certificate, but were assured that the physicians and medical examiners just didn't know what else to call it.

As the months passed, Mary read the obituary columns almost daily and heard about six to eight other families who had lost their babies in a similar manner. She wrote or called many of the mothers and began collecting newspaper and magazine articles on the Sudden Infant Death Syndrome. Through her pediatrician, Dr. Robert Polley, she learned that the Washington State Medical Association had a special committee of physicians committed to finding some answers to this problem. She learned that the committee was meeting regularly, but had no plan or particular direction.

Along with a few other concerned parents, Mary organized a meeting with these doctors. As a first step, the physicians' committee felt it was imperative to have all the infants autopsied in one central location. A problem of insufficient funds for transporting infants from different parts of the state to one place arose.

It occurred to Fred Dore that the problem could be solved through an enabling law in the state legislature. A figure of

$20,000 for the first year was projected as a realistic amount to enable the program to get off the ground. The group recognized they would need the help and support of the County Coroner, Mr. Leo Sowers, under whose jurisdiction autopsies in King County were performed. Because Senator Dore and Mr. Sowers belonged to opposing political parties, Fred felt he would have to tread very carefully and diplomatically when approaching the coroner for his support. Unknown to the Dores, Mr. Sowers and his wife had lost a baby to SIDS several years earlier and it did not take long for the two men to become allies in the effort to pass the necessary legislation.

Senator Dore set to work immediately at the state capitol in Olympia, picking up co-sponsors for his bill, which came to be designated SB180. Mr. Sowers lobbied for the legislation on the Republican side of the aisle and Senator Dore on the Democratic side. The most effective lobbying, however, was directed by Mrs. Dore and Mrs. Sowers—towards the wives of the legislators. The original bill was amended to include children up to the age of three years and the University of Washington hospital was the obvious location for the performance of the autopsies. The bill passed the State Senate, but was held up for a time in the House Rules Committee. For a time it appeared as if SB180 would die in the 1962–63 legislative session, but Fred, as Chairman of the Appropriations Committee, was able to push his bill through the Rules Committee.

On March 11, 1963, the day before the Dores' next child was born, SB180 passed the Washington State Legislature. The bill, as originally passed, directs that all babies under three years of age, dying suddenly, ". . . when in apparent good health without medical attendance with 36 hours preceding death" be autopsied through the facilities of the University of Washington School of Medicine. It requires a coroner's autopsy, "where death results from unknown or obscure causes."

Coroners throughout the state were given the jurisdiction to transport bodies of children under three years of age to the medical school for autopsy to determine the cause of death. The $20,000 appropriation passed and was to cover the cost of the autopsies. Subsequently, the location for the performance of the autopsies was moved to the Children's Orthopedic Hospital and Medical Center, a hospital affiliated with the University of Washington. Mary Dore did not confine her lobbying to legislatures or legislators' wives. Even before the bill was introduced, she descended upon the University of Washington Medical School. Her pleas fell upon receptive ears. Studies were begun by Dr. Warren Guntheroth, a pediatric cardiologist, and Dr. Donald Peterson, the epidemiologist for the Seattle/King County Health Department, who also taught at the medical school. Mary's most important convert was the Chairman of the Pediatrics Department, Dr. Robert Aldrich, who early in 1963 was designated by President John F. Kennedy to be the first Director of the newly created National Institute of Child Health and Human Development (NICHHD). When Aldrich moved to Washington, D.C. he took with him another Seattle pediatrician, Dr. Gerald LaVeck, who was to succeed Aldrich as the second director of NICHHD.

Seattle was thus the logical meeting ground for scientists from around the world to discuss the problem of the Sudden Infant Death Syndrome. NICHHD provided the funds for the meeting, which was chaired by Dr. Ralph Wedgwood, chairman of the Pediatric Department, and Dr. Earl Benditt, chairman of the Pathology Department—both of the University of Washington.

The purpose of the meeting was twofold: to examine critically what was then known about sudden death in infancy and to recommend pathways of research that needed to be explored to find definitive answers. The conference was remarkably successful in meeting both objectives; the proceedings were printed and distributed by the National Institutes of Health. SIDS research had moved from the county morgue to research laboratories. A tiny snowball had begun to roll.

An important question that could not be resolved at the 1963 conference was whether the stricken infants were victims of a single disease process or whether they were dying coincidentally of several different diseases. It was the unanimous feeling of those present that more precise studies to define both the epidemiology and pathology of sudden infant death were needed. The answers to these questions were available by the time the Second International Conference was held in 1969.

Again the Second Conference took place in Washington, this time at an old hotel in the picturesque San Juan Islands about 90 miles north of Seattle. This location was chosen so that the scientists would be free of city-life distractions and able to completely immerse themselves in the subject for two and a half days. The National Institute of Child Health and Human Development again provided funds for the conference as well as for publication of the proceedings by the University of Washington Press.

The 1969 Conference co-chairmen were Drs. Bergman and Beckwith who had come to Seattle in 1964; they were joined in editing the proceedings by a third colleague, Dr. C. George Ray, a virologist, who joined the Seattle research team in 1967. The focus of the Conference was on work that had been accomplished between 1963 and 1969.

The opening talk, Progress in Sudden Infant Death Research, 1963–69, was given, fittingly, by Dr. Marie A. Valdes-Dapena* of Philadelphia, who was accepted as the most impeccable source of scientific information on crib death.

In her talk, Dr. Dapena listed nine new theories that had been proposed to explain crib death since the 1963 conference. They were: stress, adrenal hormone imbalance, mineral imbalance, abnormal reflex of the cardio-vascular system, a deficiency of the parathyroid gland, bacterial infection, spinal cord bleeding due to "whip lash" injury, infanticide (a New York psychiatrist actually wrote a paper in 1968 suggesting that crib death was due to depressed mothers killing their babies) and obstruction of the nasal passage due to mucus. All of these proposed theories, with the exception of the

---

* "Molly" Dapena, as she's know to her colleagues, is the world's most respected authority on Sudden Infant Death Syndrome, and a most remarkable woman. Dr. Dapena has spent the past 15 years trying to unravel the mystery of crib death. In the process, she's examined and critically evaluated most of the prevailing theories about the syndrome, discarding some along the way and continuing to research others.

Dr. Dapena is an associate professor of pathology at St. Christopher's Hospital for Children in Philadelphia and teaches pediatric pathology at nearby Temple University Medical School. Married 28 years to Dr. Antonio Valdes-Dapena, Chief of Pathology at the University of Pennsylvania Graduate Hospital, the two doctors are the parents of 11 children. Dr. Antonio, in addition to being a distinguished scientist, is an accomplished linguist. Together, the two have familiarized themselves with the entire world literature devoted to SIDS. Dr. Marie has had published a number of scholarly papers on the subject, among them, a review of the world literature from 1954 through 1966, undertaken with the help of a grant from NICHHD. Dr. Dapena, busy as she is, serves as Chairwoman of the Medical Board of the National Foundation for Sudden Infant Death, Inc., as well as vice-president and trustee of the organization. The National Foundation (for SID) has maintained high standards for scientific inquiry because of the involvement of Dr. Dapena. Her reputation for integrity and the respect with which she's held by the medical community is unimpeachable.

last one (proposed by Dr. Edward Shaw of San Francisco), were convincingly disproved. Several other theories will be discussed shortly. Part of the conference was devoted to sessions on terminology and definition. One entire session was devoted to the question of terminology. Dr. Beckwith proposed the adoption of the term. Sudden Infant Death Syndrome for the phenomenon previously called crib death, cot death (in Great Britain), Sudden Unexpected Death or Sudden Unexplained Death:

> Those of us in this room have applied a great many names to this entity. Yet the terms we use are sufficiently alike that one might hope that some sort of consensus might be achieved. The need for this is perhaps self-evident. It would be a good thing indeed if, in future publications, in naming of parent groups and in discussing this with the lay press, the same name could be used.
> A good title for this entity should be short and euphonious, sufficiently descriptive to prevent confusion with other types of sudden death, and readily comprehensible to lay persons.
> Since the 1963 conference, we in Seattle have favored the term "Sudden Death Syndrome." This has the important virtue of communicating to the medical profession the concept that this is, in fact, a distinctive clinicopathological entity. The word "syndrome" also combines well with modifiers to form a collective noun and hence provides a better name for a disease entity than, for example, "Sudden Unexpected Death in Infancy." The latter is a fine name for a paper, but not for a disease. The advantages, however, are at least partially negated by the fact that the word "syndrome" is not in the vocabulary of most lay persons. I personally feel the term "Sudden Death Syndrome" should at least be amplified to include the word "infant." The reason for this is that a number of syndromes of sudden death occur at different ages, and papers entitled "Sudden Death Syndrome" alone could refer to any of these.

The popular term "Sudden Unexpected Death" has the important disadvantage of embracing unexpected death due to a variety of clearly defined diseases.

I should therefore like to cast my vote for the term "Sudden Infant Death Syndrome (SIDS)" as the best of many possible expressions for this entity.

Although this proposal was not unanimously accepted at the conference, the term "Sudden Infant Death Syndrome" has taken hold and is in general use among physicians.

Definition proved to be a far more vexing problem than terminology. Previously crib death had been a "diagnosis of exclusion," meaning that it could only be diagnosed when the possibility of all other diseases had been excluded. Considering the new evidence that had been accumulated since 1963, the seven pathologists present at the conference met separately from the rest and came forth with the criteria needed for a positive diagnosis of SIDS.

An acceptable definition of the Sudden Infant Death Syndrome was established to be "the sudden death of any infant or young child, which is unexpected by history, and in which thorough post-mortem examination fails to demonstrate an adequate cause for death."

One of the central problems was in the last clause of the definition as a "thorough post-mortem examination" was open to considerable discussion. Beckwith set forth his concept of a minimal acceptable work up:

1. Adequate history.
2. Gross examination, *including* thorax, abdomen, brain, entire larynx and spinal cord.
3. Blood culture.
4. Histological examination, including: brain, heart, lungs, liver, kidneys, and other organs as indicated by nos. 1 and 2 above.

5. Ancillary studies (toxicological, chemical, special cultures, virological studies, and so forth) as indicated by results of above.
6. Counseling of family.

After additional consideration, Beckwith's proposal was accepted with modification. It was felt that neither gross examination of the spinal cord nor blood culture, albeit desirable, would be essential for the inclusion of patients in certain studies. Crib death had become a disease.

V

DEFINING SUDDEN INFANT DEATH SYNDROME

"One of the more difficult and controversial problems in this subject is that of definition. As is often the case with diseases or syndromes, a rigid definition is neither possible nor even appropriate until the etiology and pathogenesis are understood."

J. Bruce Beckwith, M.D.
The Sudden Infant Death Syndrome
Current Problems in Pediatrics
June 1973

Crib death had finally come to be considered a disease. The remainder of the 1969 conference was devoted to sessions on its epidemiology, pathology, virology and physiology. Drawing from the basic knowledge presented at that conference, along with subsequent developments, we now turn to a description of SIDS.

EPIDEMIOLOGY

It is the function of epidemiology to describe the various outward characteristics of a disease. SIDS has remarkably consistent characteristics as ascertained by comparing studies from different parts of the world. Good epidemiologic studies have been conducted in Philadelphia, Cleveland, Seattle and San Diego in the United States; in Ontario,

Canada; Brisbane, Australia; Prague, Czechoslovakia and in Northern Ireland. Everywhere the picture is similar.

In describing the epidemiological characteristics of SIDS, the words "common," "frequent," "usually," are often used. The reader is advised to interpret them in a statistical sense. For example, SIDS is *more apt* to occur in a black premature baby at three months of age. It is *less apt* to occur in a full term white baby at eight months of age. This doesn't mean it won't happen to such a baby; it just means when the entire population of babies are taken into account, the odds make the occurrence more frequent in some than in others.

This point is stressed because of the numerous calls and letters received from parents who feel their babies may have been abnormal or "freakish" because they didn't fit into the most common pattern. Naturally a baby is an individual and not a statistical figure to his parents. Even though SIDS is rare after one year of age, it *does* occur. And to the family of the victim, the event is as real and horrible as to the family of a three-month-old victim. Statistics are valuable only when interpreted properly.

INCIDENCE

According to the epidemiologic studies mentioned above, the incidence of SIDS varies between 1.5 and 3 per 1000 live births, averaging around 2.3. This means that roughly one out of every 350 babies born into this world is destined to die of SIDS. The incidence does not appear to have changed over the years, though this is difficult to determine with certainty because SIDS was called by so many different names in the past, and still is. It is also not possible to relate the incidence in developing countries because relatively few infants who die are autopsied.

How many babies die of crib death every year in the United States? The exact number is not known since SIDS has not been a "reportable" illness as defined in the International Classification of Diseases used by vital statisticians. Furthermore, the disease is called by so many different names on death certificates, it would be impossible to collect accurate statistics. For example, a great many pathologists use the term "interstitial pneumonia" to describe a typical case; under procedures of the Bureau of Vital Statistics reporting, such cases would be entered under "Respiratory Illness, pneumonia." At the time of the 1963 conference, therefore, participants could only "guesstimate" the number of yearly cases, and that figure ranged anywhere from ten thousand to twenty-five thousand yearly in the United States.

In succeeding years, sophisticated epidemiologists turned their talents towards finding more precise answers. One of these was Donald Peterson, then epidemiologist for the Seattle-King County Health Department, and now Professor of Epidemiology at the University of Washington School of Public Health and Community Medicine. Peterson found that even if the terms "SIDS" or "crib death" did not appear on death certificates, it was still possible through circumstantial evidence to isolate the number of children in a community dying of SIDS. He did this by reviewing all infant deaths in the community between the ages of one and twelve months that did not occur in the hospital or under medical observation. He sought all stricken children who had had no prior illness and were pronounced dead at home or upon arrival at a hospital emergency room. By this method Peterson came up with the incidence figure of 3.2 per thousand live births.

How accurate was this "rough" study utilizing only death certificates instead of a personal study of each case? Several "tight" epidemiologic studies were then conducted, the most extensive being in Belfast, Northern Ireland by Doctors Peter Froggat and T. K. Marshall, and in Seattle by Doctors Bergman, Beckwith, and Ray. A "tight" study meant that every single infant death in the community was closely monitored by the study team. For instance, if a physician chose not to report a case to the coroner, signed the death certificate himself and diagnosed pneumonia, this sequence of facts was picked up through a review of all death certificates, and the physician was questioned about the circumstances of death.

The total number of cases of SIDS, then, can best be related to the number of live births in a given community. The incidence figure—between two and three per thousand live births—seems to be consistent wherever good epidemiologic studies have been done. In the past, we have used the figure ten thousand infants per year dying of SIDS in the United States. The figure was derived by multiplying every thousand babies born by the figure 2.5. Since the birth rate in the United States has dropped rapidly in the last

THE MONTHS OF BIRTH OF 309 CASES OF SIDS
IN KING COUNTY DURING SIX-YEAR PERIOD
(1965–1971) COMPARED WITH THE AVERAGE
TOTAL NUMBER OF BIRTHS BY MONTH
IN KING COUNTY IN SAME TIME PERIOD

	Months of Birth					
	Jan	Feb	Mar	Apr	May	June
SIDS Cases	29	22	14	19	18	23
Monthly Average of Total Births	1,460	1,446	1,635	1,547	1,619	1,586

	Months of Birth						
	July	Aug	Sept	Oct	Nov	Dec	Total
SIDS Cases	28	36	27	39	38	30	309
Monthly Average of Total Births	1,630	1,625	1,611	1,603	1,529	1,659	18,950

several years, the total number of deaths is now lower. In 1973 therefore, we estimate that approximately seven thousand five hundred babies will die of SIDS—still an enormous toll.

AGE DISTRIBUTION

One of the most striking and puzzling features of SIDS is the characteristic age distribution. As mentioned previously, the very youngest infants are spared. In the Seattle series of over 500 cases, the earliest that SIDS occurred was in an infant of 13 days.

SIDS is often confused with the most common affliction of the newborn period, Respiratory Distress Syndrome, also known as hyaline membrane disease. This entity is the largest cause of death in infancy which characteristically affects the breathing of tiny premature infants a few hours after birth. Incidence of SIDS, on the other hand, occurs between

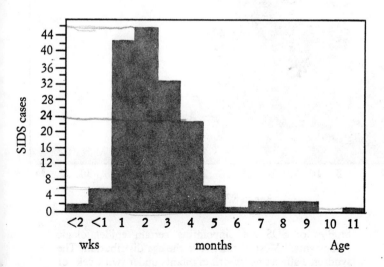

The age distribution of 1970 cases of SIDS, January 1, 1965-September 1, 1968.

10 and 16 weeks. It is rare after six months, and exceedingly rare after one year of age.

This is what Dr. Beckwith says about SIDS in the older baby:

> SIDS is a disease that most commonly strikes between two weeks and six months of age, with a peak incidence between two and three months. However, the age distribution curve is a typical bell-shaped one, with occasional cases occurring as early as the first few days of life, or beyond the age of 12 months. About ninety percent (90%) of cases occur in the first six months, with most of the remainder occurring before the first birthday. As with any entity, however, there are exceptions. 'Classic' SIDS is known to strike infants beyond the age of one year. It is particularly desirable that a complete postmortem examination be done in children over a year to

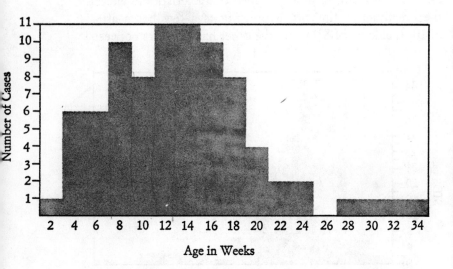

Studies of SDS are pinpointing certain epidemiologic "Constants." Most distinctive is the age distribution. The syndrome almost never strikes infants under two weeks or over eight months old. Peak incidence occurs between one and four months.

confirm the diagnosis, since the likelihood of other conditions such as heart disease or meningitis is greater in this
group. If the disease and pathological findings are com-
patible with SIDS, that diagnosis is reasonable for the rare
child that does die in the second year. Just because the
event occurs rarely, it is every bit as real to the family of
an 'older' SIDS victim as it is to the family who loses an
infant in the most frequent age group. Because the 'older'
victim has lived with his family longer, and because SIDS
literature stresses incidence in the younger age group,
grief-guilt feelings of parents may be unusually intense.
Special counseling efforts are therefore indicated to convince these parents that they were in NO way responsible
for their child's death.

SEX

About sixty percent (60%) of SIDS victims are boys as
compared to forty percent (40%) girls. The fact that males
are struck down more frequently is not unique to SIDS; it
appears in many other diseases, like infections and accidents.

SIDS in King County (Jan. 1965-Sept. 1968) by
Sex and Race Compared to Total Live Births

Race	SIDS Cases	Live Births	Rate/1000 Live Births
Males			
White	87	34,447	2.53
Black	8	1,629	4.91
Oriental	2	577	3.47
Others*	4	803	4.98
Total Males	101	37,554	2.69
Females			
White	50	32,664	1.53
Black	8	1,638	4.90
Oriental	2	577	3.47
Others*	10	828	12.08
Total Females	69	35,761	1.93
Overall rate of SIDS/1000 live births 170/73,315 = 2.32			

* Mostly Indian.

In terms of susceptibility to disease, females seem to be the stronger sex. More male babies are born into the world and more females are left inhabiting it. Though no one knows for certain the reason why, some geneticists speculate as follows: females possess two X chromosomes and males one; that is the basic biological difference between the sexes. It is thought that the X chromosome contains some protective mechanism against disease. The female, thus, would get a "double dose" of this protective material, leaving her better able to cope with the perils of our environment.

BIRTH WEIGHT

Babies born with a weight lighter than five pounds are a higher risk for SIDS; the smaller the baby, the higher the risk. There also seems to be a higher incidence of SIDS in

EPIDEMIOLOGY OF SUDDEN INFANT DEATH

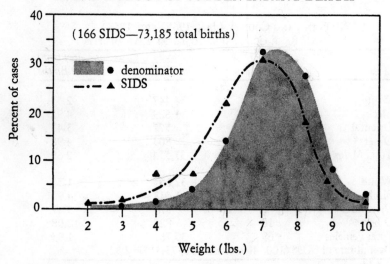

The birth weight of 166 SIDS victims compared to other children born during the same time period, January 1, 1965-September 1, 1968.

twins or triplets. Whether this is due to the fact that they are the products of a multiple pregnancy or because they are usually low birth-weight babies is not known.

SEASON

The incidence of SIDS is usually lowest during the summer months and highest during the late fall and winter. This distribution seems to coincide with the peak periods of respiratory illness in a community for both adults and children. In Australia and New Zealand, where respiratory illness coincides with the cold season in summer, SIDS is also more frequent in the summer time.

SOCIO-ECONOMIC CLASS

Infants born into privileged surroundings are not spared by SIDS. The children of two Seattle physician families died in the past year. Nevertheless, SIDS definitely occurs more

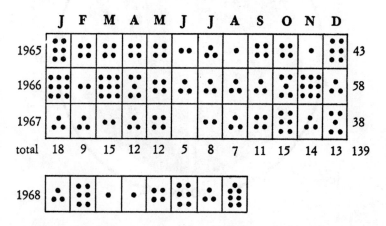

The months of death of 170 SIDS cases January 1, 1965-September 1, 1968 demonstrating seasonal variation. ● = 1 case of SIDS.

frequently in families of lower socio-economic class. The incidence is also higher among minority groups such as blacks, American Indians and Mexican Americans—not because of racial characteristics but because more of these families live in less fortunate circumstances. While the overall risk of SIDS is one in every 350 babies, the risk to a black infant in an urban ghetto is in the order of one out of 80.

Professor Josef Houstek of Charles University in Prague, has shown that SIDS correlates with infant mortality in general. Thus, in countries which have very low infant mortality rates, like Sweden and the Netherlands, SIDS is a much rarer occurrence.

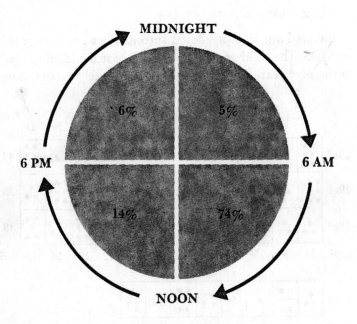

The times of day that 160 SIDS victims were discovered, January 1, 1965-Septmeber 1, 1968, coinciding with hours of sleep.

SLEEP

A distinctive feature of SIDS is that virtually every child is discovered lifeless. In the Seattle study, every single baby died during sleep. Any baby who showed signs of life and then died under observation was found at autopsy to have succumbed to some other disease. Does this mean that every baby who dies of SIDS must be asleep? No. Reputable pathologists have told us that they have studied the occasional child who died of SIDS while awake. However, the circumstance, is exceedingly rare.

We have talked with parents who thought their babies were alive when initially found. But deeper probing revealed that they mistakenly took for signs of life phenomena that occurred after death; for example, blueness of the face, open eyes without signs of motion, apparent chest movement during mouth-to-mouth resuscitation. All of these are phenomena that occur naturally *after* death.

FEEDING

A great deal of emotion often accompanies discussions about infant feeding. There also is a renewed interest in nutrition in the United States exemplified by the multimillion dollar business done by the health food industry and the enormous sale of books on nutrition and health. It is not surprising therefore, that much attention has been directed towards the possible relationship between SIDS and feeding.

Allergy to cow's milk causing crib death was a very prevalent theory in Great Britain during the 1960's and still has some support, mostly in that country. The hypothesis originally put forth by some eminent British immunologists was based on studies in rabbits. They observed that when milk was sprayed into the lungs of rabbits during sleep, a severe allergic reaction would result, terminating in death. They theorized that some babies during sleep could regurgitate milk from their stomachs that could pass into the wind pipe and cause a similar fatal reaction. What made the milk allergy theory even more promising at the time was the finding that SIDS occurred only in babies fed with cow's milk. Participants at the 1963 Seattle conference could not recall documented cases of SIDS occurring in breast-fed babies.

A nutritional explanation for crib death, was and still is, abetted by another factor: wishful thinking. Would that it were true! If only some dietary lack could be found to explain SIDS, a supplement could be added and a DREAD DISEASE COULD BE PREVENTED. But reality has an ugly way of intruding on the world of make believe. Sadly, the milk allergy theory did not hold up. As a result of research conducted in the late 1960's, it was found that the reason that fewer breast-fed babies die of crib death in the United States and the United Kingdom is that there are fewer babies fed by breast in those two countries. When a large enough population was sampled, it was found that there are wholly breast-fed babies who die of SIDS, as well as babies who are fed on goat's milk, soy milk, and other cow's milk substitutes.

Lately some scientists have raised the possibility of SIDS being due to deficiencies in certain trace elements such as magnesium, calcium, selenium and Vitamin E. No confirmation has been found for any of these theories. We will discuss the damage done by propagation of some theories in a later chapter.

SLEEPING POSITION

The possible relationship of a sleeping position is an example of how easy it is to be fooled by simple observations, without looking around to see what occurs in the normal population. In statistics this is called the importance of "normal controls." At the outset of the Seattle study it was found that most of the crib death victims had been put to sleep on their abdomens. The investigators were so struck by this observation that they began to feel that babies put to sleep on their back might be protected against crib death. They felt that way until they asked local Seattle pediatricians to sample the mothers in their practices to see how they normally laid their babies down to sleep. It was found that eighty-five percent (85%) of babies in the Seattle area were put to sleep on their abdomens or sides; less than fifteen percent (15%) were put down to sleep on their backs. When a greater number of SIDS cases had been accumulated, the same breakdowr ensued. In other words, about fifteen percent (15%) of victims were put to sleep on their back, the same percentage as in the "normal" population. Also, in Great Britain, where babies are much more commonly placed to sleep on their backs, the SIDS incidence is the same as in the United States.

CLINICAL FINDINGS

SIDS claims thin babies and fat babies, black ones and white ones, clean ones and dirty ones, those with diaper rashes and those with completely clear skin, those with colds and those in the peak of health, those who are loved and wanted, and those who are neglected and unwanted. The victims of SIDS do not show any characteristics that would distinguish them from the normal population of infants. Exhaustive studies have been done on the health of families, care and health of the mother during pregnancy, labor and delivery records, medical history during the weeks and months prior to death. Nothing that would point a finger at any particular child as a potential victim of crib death has emerged from these studies.

Just over half the babies who die seem to have slight colds, characterized by runny noses. This means that half of the victims *don't* have colds. The typical story is that the infant is put down to sleep either at night or during nap time and discovered lifeless. A characteristic finding that we feel is an extremely important part of the puzzle is the apparent *silent* nature of death. Many, many parents reported finding their babies dead while sleeping in the same room or even the same bed, without hearing the slightest sound.

Another common but not invariable finding is of apparent tumult in the bed. The baby who was laid down to sleep in the middle of the bed may be found wedged up in one corner with bedclothes in disarray. Often the bedclothes cover the face leading to the erroneous notion of suffocation.

Two other findings are extremely frightening to parents when they come upon their lifeless child. Firstly, a bloody froth often comes out through the nose, and even stains the sheets. Many parents feel this represents internal bleeding. Actually, the froth is a result of "pulmonary edema," or extra fluid that collects in the lungs and bubbles out through the wind pipe and nose. It is a characteristic feature of SIDS.

Another common finding is apparent bruising on one part of the body, leading parents to feel that the child has been injured. This disturbing sign is due to the fact that as soon as a person dies, the blood stops circulating and settles down to the deep end and portions of the body. Therefore, if the body is lying sideways and the left cheek is against the bed, a large purple mark might be expected to appear in that area.

Finally, the diaper of the baby is usually full of stool and urine, and at autopsy the urinary bladder is almost always empty. The Seattle research group used the disturbances from the original sleeping position as evidence for a very brief but active, convulsive type movement occurring just seconds prior to death.

PATHOLOGICAL OBSERVATIONS

Like most pathologists, Dr. Bruce Beckwith is a careful observer. That characteristic after all is a hallmark of a pathologist's trade; his job is to determine what in the body goes wrong to cause illness. In the early 1960's, Beckwith was training to become a pediatric pathologist under the supervision of Dr. Benjamin Landing at Children's Hospital in Los Angeles. Like many young physicians in training, his salary was small and he had a family to feed. He supplemented his income and gained valuable experience by working part-time in the office of the Los Angeles County Coroner. Because of his interest in the pathology of children, Beckwith was given virtually all of the children's work in the coroner's office, which were mostly cases of crib death. So even before coming to Seattle to embark on a formal research program in SIDS in the middle of 1964, Beckwith had already studied over four hundred cases of SIDS in the L.A. County Coroner's office. In so doing, he made an observation so fundamental that generations of future scientists may well look upon it as the turning point in understanding the mechanisms of SIDS. That observation involved the distribution of petechiae over the thymus gland.

The thymus gland, as has already been described, is a fatty organ that lies over the heart and the great vessels in the chest cavity. It is relatively large in young infants. The thymus gradually atrophies in later childhood and is only a tiny structure by adolescence and adult life. While most of the thymus gland lies in the chest cavity, a tiny part of it extends up alongside a blood vessel into the neck. Petechiae are minute red dots caused by rupture of the tiniest of blood vessels, called capillaries. These vessels can rupture from a variety of different reasons such as infection, allergy, or trauma. Pathologists had noticed the presence of petechiae over the thymus gland in SIDS cases for years but placed no particular significance on the observation.

Beckwith, on the other hand, noticed that the petechiae were not distributed evenly over the gland. There is a heavier concentration of these small red dots in the lower portion of the gland located in the chest, while the portion extending into the neck is relatively spared.

Taken by itself the observation is probably meaningless. However, there are other pathological features of interest. As mentioned previously, the urinary bladder and bowel are usually empty. The lungs are filled with a bloody fluid (pulmonary edema) causing them to weigh more than twice normal at autopsy. Interesting but nonspecific (it appears in other disorders) is the finding that the blood does not clot after death, as it usually should.

Finally, and extremely important in making a diagnosis of SIDS, no other lesion sufficient to cause death should be present on post-mortem examination. In ten to fifteen percent of babies who die suddenly and unexpectedly, an explained cause will be found other than SIDS. This is one reason it is important to obtain autopsies in all cases of sudden unexpected infant death. Other conditions that can cause infants to die suddenly and unexpectedly are overwhelming bacterial infection, inflammation of the heart muscle, and bleeding within or around the brain.

DIFFERENTIATION BETWEEN SIDS AND CHILD ABUSE

It is important at this point to bring up the subject of child abuse or, as it is more popularly called, the "battered child syndrome." Child abuse is similar to crib death in that only in recent years has the extent of the problem become known to both the medical profession and the public. Also, like SIDS, community-wide programs are required to deal with the problem; no one profession or agency can handle it alone. On the other hand, it is crucial to recognize that SIDS and the battered child syndrome are two different entities that can be readily distinguished by competent medical authorities. Parents of crib death victims have suffered through the ages from accusing fingers pointed at them. Ironically, public awareness of the battered child syndrome is making the plight of SIDS parents worse in some communities. In other words, with increasing awareness of both SIDS and the battered child syndrome, there is unwarranted confusion between these "new" phenomena, with the SIDS parent again being made to suffer even more from losing a treasured infant.

How can the two conditions be differentiated? First, the age incidence is different. Whereas SIDS peaks at three months of age, it is rare for that age infant to suffer physical abuse. In the Seattle area we see approximately sixty cases of SIDS a year, whereas *deaths* from child abuse number less than eight. Finally, and most important, a competent pathologist can easily tell the difference. There are characteristic findings on the autopsy of the child who has been traumatized, both externally and internally. They are not found in SIDS. Again, the two problems are important but very different, and should not be confused.

ISOLATION OF VIRUSES

It has been suspected by many workers since the pioneering observations of Werne and Garrow that infectious agents played a significant role in SIDS. The epidemiologic data most resemble that seen in acute viral illnesses. The age distribution, seasonality, and increased number of babies with colds all support the idea. Pathological evidence includes inflammatory changes all along the respiratory tract. Infectious agents have been prime suspects. But which ones?

Energetic searches have been made for bacteria without success. Scientists have also searched for viruses but they are technically more difficult to isolate than bacteria. Dr. C. George Ray in Seattle, and Dr. Carl Brandt in Washington, D.C., utilizing newer techniques in the middle 1960's, were successful in isolating viruses from babies who died of SIDS.

Ray's "new technique" is interesting to describe. Because viruses need special culture medium to grow, specimens are usually taken and stored in freezers until a number of them can be planted on culture medium at the same time. Ray, however, planted his specimens immediately and profited by a higher isolation rate. The explanation is that the viruses were probably destroyed by the freezing process. In any case, Ray found potentially harmful viral agents in just over a third of SIDS cases as compared with a sixth of control cases. The viruses he isolated were not strange or particularly virulent ones; they were the same ones that cause common colds.

Though viruses of the upper respiratory tract probably do play an important role in most cases, they probably do so as a "trigger agent" rather than a causal one. The viral component is receiving increased research attention not because it is an entire answer to the puzzle of SIDS, but rather because it is approachable from a therapeutic and preventative standpoint.

The fact that viruses are isolated from only a third of SIDS cases does not mean that the agents are absent in the other two thirds. The tiny organisms are simply too difficult to isolate even in diseases like encephalitis that are known to be caused by viruses. While there is no reason to think that viruses must be present in *every* case of SIDS, we feel they play a contributory though not causal role.

THE CAUSE OF SIDS

As the reader now well knows, the cause of SIDS is not known. There have been many theories put forward to explain the strange disease, some of which have been discussed in earlier pages. Hundreds of letters have come to the authors from persons all over the world with ideas about the cause and prevention of SIDS. Some are frivolous, some are ugly, but most are entirely sincere and represent a genuine desire to help with a tragic problem. Because the authors are so heavily involved in the "human" aspects of SIDS, we rather arbitrarily classify theories as "benign" or "wicked." The latter, of course, would be those that augment the already present guilt in families by charging that SIDS could have been prevented by some action of the parent.

Some of the more recently espoused theories will be discussed here. Suffocation, still a recurring theory, has already been dealt with—sufficiently, we hope, to banish it forever from the reader's mind.

COW'S MILK ALLERGY

The authors, from the perspectives of a pediatrician and mother respectively, both wholeheartedly endorse breast feeding for young infants. The reason is that if the mother is comfortable with the idea, the experience can be a beautiful one for both mother and child. If the mother is not comfortable about breast feeding she should have no pangs of guilt; bottle feeding is completely satisfactory. Our endorsement of breast milk is *not* however because it bears any possible relationship to SIDS.

ENDOCRINE INSUFFICIENCY

Some scientists were attracted to the idea that a deficiency of some hormone like that produced from the adrenal gland was responsible for SIDS. Studies of the last five years, however, have shown that there is no glandular abnormality noted at autopsy and the hormone level in the blood stream is the same for babies who die of SIDS and those who succumb to other diseases.

A Danish physician, Preban Geertinger, wrote a book about SIDS and suggested that the disease was due to an insufficiency of a tiny gland called the parathyroid. He based this on his inability to find this gland in a third of SIDS cases, and postulated that this may be in some way related to Vitamin D deficiency in the mother. However convincing this sounded in theory, it was not borne out by the facts. Dr. Valdes-Dapena was able to find the parathyroid gland in all cases of SIDS that she studied. Furthermore, low serum calcium levels, the result of Vitamin D deficiency, have not been detected in victims of SIDS.

A great many letters we receive concern the possibility that SIDS is caused by chemicals or toxins present in our "modern society." A whole host of these have been suggested—detergents, bleach, flouride, air pollution, to name just a few. All of these toxic theories would be ruled out by both the epidemiology and the pathology findings. Also, SIDS seems to have been present many years before these products came into common use.

HEART DEFECT

When any person dies, two things happen. The lungs stop breathing and the heart stops beating. In SIDS, which comes first? This question is still debated vigorously among scientists interested in the disease. At the time of the 1963 Conference, there was roughly a fifty-fifty split among those attending, as to whether the death in SIDS was primarily cardiac or respiratory. By the time of the Second Conference in 1969, the majority opinion held that the death was primarily a respiratory one. However, decisions on scientific matters are not made by majority vote, and strong advocates of a cardiac mechanism of death still exist.

IMMUNE DEFECT

Newborn babies are endowed from their mothers with protective material in their blood to ward off infections. This fraction of the blood is called gamma globulin. As the mother's gift of gamma globulin begins to wear out, the baby starts producing its own. The point where the maternal antibody is lowest and when the baby's production mechanism is still slow is at three months of age. The fact that the peak incidence of SIDS is also at this age has sent immunologists scurrying to try to find some defect in the protective mechanism of babies who die of SIDS. Immunoglobin levels have been studied by a number of investigators without any abnormality being detected in babies who die of SIDS. They continue to search.

BLOCKED NASAL PASSAGE

Dr. Edward Shaw, a distinguished pediatrician from San Francisco, has put forth an intriguing "blocked nose" theory.

Certain babies, Shaw observes, are "obligatory nose breathers." This means that even when their noses become stuffy, they simply will not open their mouths to breathe. There is a very rare congenital defect where babies are born with a blockage of their nasal passages. If such babies do not open their mouths to breathe, they die. Shaw hypothesizes a similar situation occurring in older babies whose noses become plugged with mucus. He suggests that if the baby does not open its mouth to breathe, this sets in motion a reaction causing the child's death. While the idea has not gained a great deal of support, neither has it been totally refuted. The theory is amenable to testing—a possibility in the next several years.

SPASM OF THE VOCAL CORDS

This book is not the place to present a scientific theory in any detail, but only to inform the reader about the type of thinking that is going on among medical scientists about SIDS. The interested reader will be able to find a great deal more information in the scientific literature. References to pertinent studies are included at the end of this book. Nevertheless, since one of the authors is a member of the Seattle research team, a brief description of that group's theory would seem to be in order.

Mention was made in the discussion of pathologic findings about Beckwith's observation on the distribution of petechiae in the chest cavity. What is the significance of that finding? Beckwith first proposed in 1965 that the *only way* that this unusual distribution of petechiae could be produced would be through increased negative intrathoracic pressure against a closed airway. In simpler language, the phenomenon is produced by the baby's breathing muscles pulling hard but no air entering the lungs because of a tight block-

Summary Statement

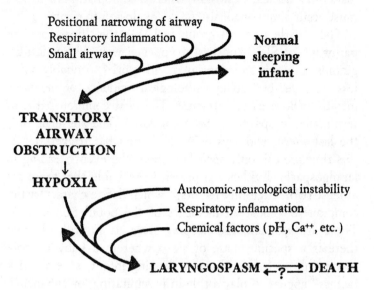

Proposed theory of Seattle investigators showing the final common pathway of SIDS terminating in laryngospasm.

age. Where would that blockage be? Remember that the baby is thought to undergo a *brief silent struggle* while asleep. The silent nature of the death suggests that the blockage is at the level of the vocal cords. It is suggested that the cords go into a spasm, close shut, and therefore cannot make any sound.

Most babies sleep with their heads turned to one side and given the presence of a slight inflammation in the airway, a movement of the head may obstruct the airway, resulting in what we have termed a laryngospasm. Dr. Beckwith has characterized SIDS as a "final common pathway," through which many babies cycle in and out, with only a few dying. He has compared this final common pathway to the "critical mass" in a nuclear explosion, where a combination of factors must occur simultaneously for the explosion to occur.

The Seattle research group feel that the "final common pathway" of SIDS consists of upper airway obstruction beginning suddenly and associated with a brief, probably noiseless struggle, producing pathological evidence of increased intrathoracic negative pressure. The final common pathway terminates in spasm of the vocal cords. The spasm is only the last event, and says nothing about what triggers it. At this time we can only speculate about the events leading to laryngospasm. Evidence is presently available that there are at least two "eligibility factors," which define characteristics common to almost all members of the population at risk. These are *age*, and the *sleeping state*. It is probable that there is a specific phase of sleep wherein a baby is more susceptible to SIDS. Given a sleeping infant, several "risk factors" appear to play a role in precipitating, or enhancing, the tendency towards laryngospasm. These factors are relatively nonspecific and act to make the child more susceptible either independently or interacting with other risk factors. The most apparent risk factor seems to be a minor viral upper respiratory illness. There are doubtless other risk factors of which we are not now aware.

Low birth weight is another eligibility factor. A recent finding by Naeye that the pulmonary arteries of SIDS victims are thickened, similar to those found in persons living at high altitudes, suggests that these babies may have suffered bouts of hypoxemia prior to death. Steinschneider has proposed that certain babies with a predisposition to sleep apnea, might, under certain conditions (e.g., viral infection), succumb to SIDS. Current studies in developmental sleep neurophysiology (Los Angeles) and SIDS in infant monkeys (Seattle) should provide further important clues, as there are doubtless other factors of which we are not now aware.

Because of the possible relationship to sleep apnea, the question has been raised as to whether SIDS might be prevented through use of electronic monitoring devices. It cannot be stressed too strongly that, at present, there is no evidence to support the idea that these devices can prevent SIDS. Much more research is required to discover whether it is possible to detect "susceptible" infants, and if this is achieved, to determine whether monitoring devices can, in fact, prevent the dreaded event.

In summary, a great deal has been learned in the past decade about SIDS. Probably the greatest advance has been the confirmation that SIDS is a real disease entity that can be positively diagnosed. The mechanism of death appears to be a respiratory one, whereby the vocal cords in susceptible infants suddenly snap shut during sleep closing off the airway. A viral upper-respiratory illness appears to play a role in most cases, but how it acts is not known. The two possibilities are, through irritating the vocal cords itself, or through changing the "sensitivity" of the nerve that control the opening and closing of the vocal cords. The type of child susceptible to this devastating reaction is not at all known. This subject occupies the SIDS researchers of the 1970's.

VI

THE SEATTLE-KING COUNTY SUDDEN INFANT DEATH SYNDROME STUDY

"Where would we all be without the work of those doctors in Seattle?"

SIDS Parent
September 1972

The Seattle-King County study sponsored by the National Institute of Child Health and Human Development was launched in January 1965 with a view towards meeting some of the objections raised by previous studies. Through the enabling legislation passed by the Washington State Legislature, it became possible to have all cases of sudden and unexpected death autopsied at the Children's Orthopedic Hospital and Medical Center. The study took on a multifaceted approach to include various aspects of the problem.

All babies suspected of dying of SIDS in the Seattle-King County area were brought to the Children's Hospital and autopsied by Dr. Beckwith. Dr. Beckwith also served as a deputy medical examiner for the county. (Sudden infant death is automatically a "coroner's case.") Immediately upon completion of the autopsy, Dr. Beckwith telephoned the parents to explain his findings and answer their inevitable questions. After several days each family was visited by the project nurse, Mrs. Margaret Pomeroy, R.N., who obtained

clinical information and provided counseling for the family.
Further assistance was offered to all the families by the
Washington Association for Sudden Infant Death Study, a
group of parents who had previously lost babies to SIDS.
Families presenting special problems, such as severe depression, were visited by Dr. Bergman in his role as the project
pediatrician. Though the home investigations were carried
on only until September 1968, autopsies and other laboratory studies on all cases of suspected SIDS in King County
continue.

Each case was carefully catalogued and to this date (September 1973) more than 500 cases have been studied. Results have been published in the medical literature and the
lay press from time to time, but briefly: of the 500 infant
deaths studied, 425 were left "unexplained" by post-mortem
examination. In the remaining 75, a lethal defect sufficient
to cause death was found. Occasionally, subsequent laboratory findings revealed such things as a previously unsuspected genetic disease which the parents would be told
about. Dr. Beckwith would inform the parents of the later
findings and these cases would be taken out of the SIDS
category and re-classified, though for counseling purposes,
they would remain in the SIDS group.

As with earlier studies, the age distribution was quite distinctive. The disease almost never occurs in infants under
two weeks or over eight months of age, with the peak incidence between one and four months. Whenever a case of
apparent SIDS occurred outside the two week to eight
month range, the study team suspected that SIDS was not
involved and generally those suspicions proved to be correct.

Throughout the years of the investigation, cases of SIDS
tended to occur in time-space clusters, suggestive of "micro-
epidemics." The Seattle study, along with others, demonstrated a clear-cut seasonal distribution, predominantly in

CAUSES OF DEATH AFTER ONE WEEK OF AGE KING COUNTY,
WASHINGTON DURING FIVE-YEAR PERIOD 1965–1970

Cause	Number	Percentage
1 Week—11 Months		
Total Deaths	609	
SIDS	272	45
Congenital Malformations	123	20
Diseases of Early Infancy	70	11
Influenza and Pneumonia	59	10
Accidents	39	6
All other Causes	46	8
1 Week—14 Years		
Total Deaths	1,334	
Accidents	336	25
SIDS	272	20
Congenital Malformations	198	15
Malignant Neoplasms	110	8
Influenza and Pneumonia	79	6
All other Causes	339	25

late autumn, winter and spring with a corresponding decrease in the summer months.

At the time we began to make home investigations, as part of the overall study, we were shocked and dismayed at the severe psychological disorientation suffered by so many of the parents. Earlier published studies had cited the guilt and self-incrimination which is an inevitable result of a sudden infant death. The degree of emotional trauma in the families we have spoken to, we referred to as the "psychiatric toll of SIDS." There are 8-10,000 victims of crib death in the United States each year. Each year there are that many more surviving families left to cope with the tragedy. Despite increased medical knowledge and public awareness, the psychiatric toll is enormous. The situation is intensified by the characteristic failure of a post-mortem examination to provide a satisfactory explanation for the death. In these highly charged circumstances, a careless remark about "suffocation" or "smothering" can prove devastating. Interfamilial accu-

sations, self-recrimination, and overwhelming guilt feelings
are not only frequent, but commonplace. Because of the
suddenness of such a death, parents are totally unprepared
to deal with the tragedy. Whether they verbalize it or not,
virtually all parents losing a child to crib death feel responsible. If a babysitter, grandparent or sibling discovered the
dead child, the situation becomes even more delicate. Blaming relatives and "friends" serves only to emphasize the hidden self-blame and suspicion which is already nearly too
much for the parents to bear.

In most areas of the country, SIDS falls within the jurisdiction of those whose basic orientation is to search for
signs of foul play. When an infant is found dead in its crib,
the frantic parents usually telephone for assistance from
police or fire department rescue units. Usually the child is
rushed to the emergency room of the nearest hospital where
it is pronounced dead. Grief-stricken and shocked parents
are next faced with the "routine" questioning from the legal
authorities. Whether or not an autopsy is ordered is often
left to the discretion of the local medical examiner or coroner. Occasionally insistent parents and/or physicians can
influence that decision one way or the other. Unfortunately,
in only about half the communities in the United States are
autopsies performed routinely on SIDS victims. In many
areas, an autopsy is viewed synonymously with the commission of a crime, both by the legal authorities and in the
public mind. If parents want an autopsy performed, it is
not uncommon for them to be told it is unnecessary because,
"it won't show anything anyway." While that may be essentially correct, our study in King County indicated that the
performance of a post-mortem can go a long way to relieve
some of the guilt and anxiety in parents' minds.

The grief reaction of parents has been well-described.
Briefly the initial reaction is one of shock and disbelief, fol-

lowed by a considerable testing of reality. Parents, and mothers particularly, will often speak of the dead child in a combination of past and present tenses. It is not uncommon for mothers to continue to draw the child's bath or prepare his food. A fear of going insane is often expressed. Parents report experiencing strange visceral sensations, such as "pressure in the head," "heartache" and "stomach pains." These sensations are often accompanied by a sad expression, sighing, an inability to concentrate except for the briefest periods, insomnia and excessive activity such as sweeping floors. Many express a fear of being alone. One young mother sat on a tree stump in her backyard when no one was at home, for fear of being alone in the house where the baby died. When they don't have strong business or family ties where they had been living, families often move to other homes or even other communities. Feelings of helplessness and anger are other common reactions. The anger is often directed at well-meaning friends, relatives and neighbors. Parents are fearful, particularly about the safety of their surviving children. ("I don't want the responsibility of my other children, but I can't let them out of my sight.") Because the family is in great turmoil, even the youngest toddler is aware of the upheaval. He may not be able to verbalize his fears but they are real nonetheless. He may harbor fears. ("The baby was taken away, maybe I'll be taken too.") An older child, already having trouble adjusting to the presence of a new baby, may have secretly wished that the baby would go away. When the baby dies, he often suffers severe guilt and blames himself for the baby's death.

Parents suffer further anxiety regarding any decision to have another child. And once they have made the decision, it is not uncommon for some women to have a great deal of difficulty in becoming pregnant again. If they do choose to have more children. we have tried to reassure them that there is no greater chance for SIDS to happen again in their family than in anyone else's. To view it in a more positive light, we have told them that if one of 350 babies will die, then certainly 349 will live. Most families in the King County study have had subsequent children and every one has felt the same apprehension, worry, and near panic during the first few months of the new baby's life. They are advised to *try* to avoid being overprotective and making an emotional cripple out of the next child. As Carolyn Szybist pointed out in her pamphlet, *The Subsequent Child*, "Parents of subsequent children are inclined to view the common cold with more alarm than open heart surgery." In terms of effective counseling, low-income and minority families are a particular problem. Crib deaths are more likely to occur in this group and poor housing and illegitimacy often may compound their feelings of guilt. Such families tend to be less verbal about their feelings and at the same time are less likely to have their own private physicians to help them cope with their grief.

Parents torture themselves, sometimes for years, with questions about how the death might have been avoided. When pneumonia or a similar term is used on a death certificate, the implication is left in parents' minds that the child had a demonstrable illness, with symptoms that they (or the family physician) must have missed.

SIDS may serve as the focus for parental guilt feelings about the child, particularly if the baby had been unwanted or unplanned, punished or left to cry. The universal cry of these parents is, "What did I do wrong?" In the Seattle home investigations, it became necessary to uncover the specific point around which the guilt reaction was centered and then to reassure the parents that this factor could not possibly have killed their child. Many parents need continuing reassurance on their lack of culpability.

Information Offered to Parents of SIDS Victims

1. SIDS cannot be predicted; there is no sound or cry of distress.
2. It is not preventable; death occurs during sleep.
3. The cause is unknown.
4. The cause is *not* suffocation, aspiration or regurgitation. A study by Wooley has shown that covering the faces of babies with blankets does not result in anoxemia.
5. A minor illness, such as a common cold, may often precede death.
6. There is no suffering; death probably occurs within seconds.
7. SIDS is not contagious in the usual sense. Although a viral infection may be involved, it is not a "killer virus" that threatens other family members or neighbors. SIDS rarely occurs after 6 months of age.
8. SIDS is not hereditary.
9. The baby is not the victim of a "freakish disease." From 7.5–10,000 babies die of SIDS every year in the United States.
10. SIDS is at least as old as the Old Testament and seems to have been at least as frequent in the 18th and 19th centuries as it is now. This demonstrates that new environmental agents, such as birth control pills, flouride in the water supply and detergents, do not cause SIDS. The incidence of SIDS is not rising.
11. SIDS occurs in the best of families. We have seen it happen in the hospital in infants admitted for minor surgery. (This point is especially comforting to young mothers who may feel inadequate in caring for their infants.)

Enlarged thymus

VII

DEVELOPMENT OF
THE PARENT GROUP

"All these studies convinced me that an answer could be found, would be found. But it seemed to me it would be found faster if there were some way of coordinating the efforts, some center for the exchange of information about sudden death and some public support for getting at the cause of it."

E. Jedd Roe, Jr.
REDBOOK Magazine
November 1963

To each family losing a baby suddenly and unexpectedly, the tragedy seems an isolated incident—one that affects them only. Until the formation of the Mark Addison Roe Foundation in 1962, each death was indeed isolated. Families had no one to turn to; no one had begun to estimate the extent of the problem; no one yet understood the psychological damage now associated with SIDS—no one cared.

Although the Roe Foundation was established to "promote, stimulate and support research in the diagnosis, treatment and cure of sudden, unexpected death in infants," its founders also hoped to establish a central location for families to turn to for information and assistance. The other parent organizations that followed were generally created to serve specific communities or to sponsor specific research projects. We will tell the story of one organization.

Why did parents who had lost children find it necessary to create foundations, guilds or research memorials? Why wasn't this just another disease falling within the realm of existing public institutions? Why was there no one to turn to? Rather than first chronicle the development of one parent group, it will be necessary to use hindsight to set forth the situation as it was in 1962 which, for the most part, exists today.

Unlike all other diseases, and most particularly those of childhood, the Sudden Infant Death Syndrome stands alone for one reason: it is the only known disease which is categorized into the legal system and which is almost never observed in hospitals and clinics. It is this reason, more than any other, that intensifies the guilt and grief for the surviving family members.

When illness strikes or when a heart attack kills, one turns to medical science for the answer. Hospitals, nursing homes or the doctor himself, stand by the family. If the illness is terminal, everything known to medical science is done to prolong life.

When SIDS strikes, there are no hospitals, nursing homes or doctors. There is only a vault in the morgue. There is no kindly reassurance from the medical community, only questions from legal authorities. There are no huge hospital bills to pay, only the price of a tiny coffin.

Certain classes of unexpected, unattended and unexplained deaths always fall under the jurisdiction of the legal system in all states. SIDS generally falls within this category. What happens to the victim and his family very much depends on the existing legal system as well as the person directly in charge of it. Before discussing the medico-legal problems related to the Sudden Infant Death Syndrome, it is important to examine, the two medico-legal investigative systems most frequently in practice in the United States.

Medical examiner systems exist in major urban areas or as statewide operations. This system is usually headed by a Chief Medical Examiner who has been appointed by a community board or by the highest state or local elected official. It is a non-political appointment usually held by a forensic pathologist (occasionally it will be a Board certified pathologist) with outstanding credentials. He is a physician who is knowledgeable in both pathology and law and can determine and analyze the cause of death for a court of law, through post-mortem examination and "at the scene" investigation.

Coroner systems are the most widely used systems in the United States, and they are subject to far wider differences than the medical examiner system. For the most part, coroners are not physicians and are elected by the populace in a general election. They can also be appointive positions. Anyone choosing to do so may campaign for the job. In many areas of the country, the coroner's job is handled by either the sheriff's office or the local funeral director. Most coroners have the expertise of hospital or university affiliated pathologists at hand; but some have little or no assistance in determining the cause of death. There are notable exceptions whereby forensic pathologists serve as coroners.

No matter which system exists—medical examiner or coroner—both must produce the same end result: determination of whether or not a crime has been committed. It is the decision of the legal authorities whether a specific case will be investigated, the body viewed at the scene of death or an autopsy performed. Cases which are properly investigated only constitute a tiny part of all medico-legal cases and usually occur in large metropolitan areas operating under a system having a forensic pathologist in charge. Emphasis is put on those cases which may result in trials, with the cost of investigation borne by the judicial authorities.

Usually crib deaths are not high priority items in either system. In fact, they fall relatively low on the list of cases to be investigated. There are, of course, exceptions in localities where there is an adequate budget or where the chief investigator has an interest in the problem. In jurisdictions operating with minimal budgets, crib death investigation and autopsy is almost completely eliminated. Since SIDS has not been given a code number in the International Classification of Diseases (coding has been assured for the 1975 edition), even those cases investigated and/or autopsied may be listed as any number of recognized causes of death, i.e., viral pneumonia, aspiration, accidental suffocation, so that, statistically, an accurate number of deaths cannot be obtained, and families are given implausible diagnoses to please the Bureau of Vital Statistics.

A method of dealing with an SIDS case almost completely rests on the type of system in existence and the person in charge of medico-legal investigations in each individual community. The family might be investigated or they might be ignored. They might face a coroner's inquest or they might receive a letter of sympathy and explanation from the investigating authority. They might have a thorough autopsy performed at no charge, they might have an inadequate autopsy performed at a cost, or they may have no autopsy at all. If an autopsy is performed, the family might get the preliminary results within 48 hours or they may never be told why their baby died.

To better elucidate the problem, let us examine some actual cases.

1. Three month old Jimmy Jones was discovered lifeless in his crib at 7 A.M. His father had already left for work. Mrs. Jones called the Emergency Rescue Squad which arrived in minutes and rushed Jimmy to the

local hospital emergency room. The call to the Emergency Rescue Squad had gone out over the police call system so that while resuscitation was attempted on Jimmy, a detective from the homicide squad arrived to "talk" to Mrs. Jones. "Did you drop the baby? Why didn't you take him to the doctor? Why is your pediatrician so far away from your home? Did you want the baby? Are you married? Where's your husband? Do you know how we feel about child abuse?" All this, and Jimmy had yet to be pronounced dead.

Mr. Jones arrived at the hospital as the physician pronounced Jimmy dead. The detective stopped questioning the now hysterical mother and turned his attention to the newly arrived father. "Does your wife normally abuse the baby? Why weren't you home? Etc." At no time did any hospital authority intercede on behalf of the family. The Joneses gave autopsy permission and the detective indicated that he would be most interested in the outcome.

A week later, the Jones had heard nothing. The baby's pediatrician had told them that he probably died of "flash pneumonia" and that they shouldn't worry. Three weeks went by and Mrs. Jones called the Medical Examiner's office for information. She was told that the results were still pending. After six months of constant telephone calls, a cause of death was produced: viral pneumonia. When Mrs. Jones asked how it could have been pneumonia when her husband had given the baby a bottle at 5 A.M. and he had been fine, the medical examiner's secretary answered, "Oh, don't worry about that, we usually put that down when the Doc doesn't find anything else."

2. Jane Smith was discovered dead by her parents during her afternoon nap. She was rushed to the local hospital fifteen miles away, by her father, where she was pronounced "dead on arrival." The hospital informed Mr. Smith that the baby probably died of some form of virus. A call went out to the local funeral director who immediately took the body. The sheriff's office sent a man to the hospital and he was also told that the baby probably died of a virus. The baby was buried. There was no investigation, and her parents were left with many doubts about the cause of death. When they asked health professionals about it, they were simply told that killer viruses are around and they probably took the baby out when they shouldn't have.

3. Baby Doe was found dead in his car bed by his mother while riding to visit his grandparents. She immediately hailed a police car and had the baby rushed to the nearest hospital where he was pronounced "dead on arrival." The emergency room nurse explained that the baby would have to be autopsied, to which Mrs. Doe agreed. The autopsy report was given to the Does before the funeral with a preliminary reading of "Sudden Death at Infancy." Their name was also given to the local parent group by the medical examiner's office. Within a few days of the baby's death, the Does had received a letter of sympathy and some informative material from the parent group and were given the names of other families in their area to whom they could talk.

Later in the book we will discuss systems which we consider to be excellent as well as systems which barely function. The medico-logical system must, for the most part, carry the brunt of the anguish suffered by families. These authorities tend to overlook the fact that although the "patient" is dead, the survivors are quite alive and in desperate need of sympathetic understanding and a rational explanation for the death. Even though we realize that most jurisdictions have insufficient financial and personnel resources, the time and money necessary for the development of a humane system is minimal. It could be done with little effort. As it now stands, the only thing all SIDS families have in common is the fact that they must bury their babies.

Since crib deaths are part of a system which deals with accidents, criminal acts, and legal investigation, it is understandable that to the general community this type of death is suspect. If those in authority doubt a family, it only follows that friends, neighbors and relatives will question the death as well, particularly when that death has no explanation or at least none that is readily understood.

Less than 50 years ago, parents had every reason to expect that one or more of their children would die during childbirth or infancy. As the major childhood diseases were conquered and modern medicine seemed to develop cures for everything, the infant mortality rate dropped considerably. By the 1950's, it was generally accepted that babies didn't die and that those who suffered an illness would be saved by modern medical techniques.

Therefore, the death of an apparently healthy infant brings forth a tremendous burst of theorizing on the ability of the parents to take care of and provide for their family. Everything from charges of child abuse to dismay about the use of synthetic fabrics in the crib are hurled at the family—all during a period of time when the parents (and the mother, particularly) are feeling responsible for a death which they also cannot understand.

While the general public can be forgiven its ignorance, the inability of the medical professions to see the magnitude of the problem has been inexcusable. Until recently, the syndrome had been ignored by the scientific research community, the practicing physician, and members of all health professions. As infuriating as this denial is, there is a basic cause which again goes back to the fact that these babies are part of the medico-legal system.

SIDS babies die at home. They are not seen in hospitals or university affiliated teaching institutions where most modern research is established. Pathologists, neonatalogists and related researchers who usually function in these institutions will almost never see a crib death. Babies who are brought to the hospital emergency room will either be sent on to the county morgue, if an autopsy is ordered, or to the funeral director. Neither of these settings is generally associated with biomedical research.

Academicians who write the textbooks used in medical education, again, do not know of the existence of these infants. Accordingly, medical and nursing students are not prepared for the fact that they will have to deal with a major cause of infant deaths about which they have never heard. Nor are they prepared to deal with a SIDS family arriving in the hospital emergency room with a dead infant.

More so than any other disease, the Sudden Infant Death Syndrome is a silent killer, so silent that to the medical community it has not existed. The babies die, are buried, and become numbers in some incorrect vital statistics log. Only their families remember them. With the prevailing ignorance of 1962, it was left to the families to make sure that their babies would not be forgotten. Having lost their baby, perhaps they could do something that would save other babies, other families. Maybe their grandchildren could be protected from this silent killer.

It was the need of the victim families to insure the memory of their babies that created the bond of the parent group. If medicine wouldn't help, if the general population was apathetic, if no one would attempt to answer the question "Why did my baby die", then it became necessary for the families themselves to focus attention on the problem and to guarantee that their babies did not die in vain.

THE NATIONAL FOUNDATION
FOR SUDDEN INFANT DEATH, INC.

To our knowledge, there are four organizations in the United States dealing specifically with the Sudden Infant Death Syndrome. They are: The Guild for Infant Survival (Baltimore, Md.), The Andrew Menchell Infant Survival Foundation (New York, New York), The Sudden Infant Death Research Association (Austin, Texas) and the National Foundation for Sudden Infant Death, Inc. All of these parent groups have committed themselves to solving the problem. However, our long association has been with the latter organization and it is that story we will tell in detail.

Jedd and Louise Roe had no reason to expect a tragedy to occur as they settled into a life of privilege in the summer of 1958. Jedd worked in an investment house in New York City and Louise spent her days tending their two sons in an affluent Connecticut suburb. Everything was just as they had hoped it would be.

On an October morning in 1958, six-month-old Mark Addison Roe was found dead in his crib. At the insistence of his pediatrician, an autopsy was performed. Cause of death: Acute bronchial pneumonia. Case closed.

For Mark's parents the case was only beginning. Two weeks before his death, Mark had been pronounced "normal" by his pediatrician on a well-baby check up. He had been a full-term baby and received the best of care. There was no indication of future problems. Why then did he die?

It was this question that occupied the Roes for the next three years. For Louise, there was the fear that Mark would be a small memory for her alone. For Jedd, there was the desire to try to prevent deaths like Mark's from re-occurring. The first few months after Mark's death were spent trying to sort out the isolation and guilt. It was all so inexplicable and no one could even begin to give them an answer. What had they done wrong?

It was during these months that they began to hear of others who had lost babies in the same mysterious way. Friends and acquaintances told of their own losses. Newspaper obituaries listed case after case of infants found dead in their cribs. Slowly, the isolation lifted and the sense that Mark's death was not a solitary incident led Jedd to begin the search for a foundation or a research project to which he might contribute a substantial insurance policy given Mark, by his grandfather, at birth.

By early 1962, Jedd's quest had led him to every physician who had done any scientific research into sudden unexpected infant deaths. They were few, they were scattered, and they disagreed on everything but a few minor facts. He found no foundation or project in which he and Louise could participate or establish a memorial to Mark. So, he began to investigate the possibilities of forming a foundation himself, one which would serve as a clearing house for physicians and families, and organize and support research —one that "would help solve the problem."

At the same time, a comprehensive epidemiological study on crib death was being carried out under the auspices of Dr. Milton Helpern, then Chief Medical Examiner of New York City. Under the direction of Dr. Renate Dische, the study would attempt to investigate every case of sudden, unexpected and unexplained infant death occurring in New York City with home visits, parent/physician interviews, and thorough post-mortem examination. After talking to Dr. Dische, Jedd was convinced of the importance of his cause as well as the necessity of forming a foundation to further research and understanding.

In August of that year, the Mark Addison Roe Foundation was incorporated in the state of Connecticut. It had as its trustees Jedd and Louise Roe; Dr. Dische, Mark Roe's pediatrician, J. Frederick Lee, M.D.; and Lowell Weicker, Jr., a Greenwich, Connecticut attorney (now United States Senator) and a close friend of the Roes. It had as its medical advisors Doctors Rustin McIntosh and William Silverman of the prestigious Babies Hospital in New York. There was no office and no staff. It was funded by the insurance policy, contributions from friends and relatives and the Roes themselves. The foundation would be small and "every cent would be directly put to work on the problem."

For the first five years of its existence, the foundation remained much as it had been envisioned. The primary concentration was on the Grants to Research Program through which funds were channeled to assist on-going research projects. The most notable grants were given to Dr. Marie A. Valdes-Dapena, Dr. Dische, and Dr. Daniel Stowens. Dr. Dapena herself played a great part in the early development of the foundation, particularly in its strong, careful grant review system.

Two major developments occurred at the end of the fourth year which would eventually overtake the original importance placed on the grant program. In late 1966, the first chapter of the Roe Foundation was chartered covering Nassau and Suffolk counties in New York. A special emphasis was placed on the role of public education. During this same period, the foundation and its medical advisors, now led by Dr. Dapena, developed the Common Reporting Form for Sudden Infant Death which would aid research in finding new clues as to the cause. It was to be the major contribution made by the foundation.

The form was a relatively complete pre- and post-natal history of the victim, a simple family medical history, as well as a socio-economic record. The forms were to be filled out by the attending physician or medical examiner in consultation with the parents as soon as possible after the death. Much time and money were expended on these forms. A bio-statistician was hired to compile, process and evaluate them. Preliminary distribution was done and then—the forms were eliminated on the recommendation of the Roe Foundation medical advisors.

Although the form had excellent therapeutic value to the family and could have elicited some good results, the foundation could not prepare or establish an acceptable distribution and retention plan. To receive usable data, the forms would, firstly, have had to be distributed to *every* SIDS family in a given number of communities (which would vary in geography and socio-economic levels) and, secondly, completed by a group of trained interviewers. It was a project that would have required far greater financial resources than the Mark Addison Roe Foundation possessed at that time.

While the foundation continued to operate under the guidance of the Roes, others volunteered their time and resources and began to play a role in the growth and direction of the fledgling organization. Some were other parents who had suffered similar tragedies. Some were friends who were moved by the suffering they saw. Chapters continued to develop and soon people from other areas of the country began to move the foundation into a more national front.

In 1967, the Roes moved their family to Denver, Colorado. They had arranged for office space in the basement of a Greenwich law firm but Ann and Arthur Siegal offered office space in their firm in New York City. Their offer was accepted and the foundation moved to New York City, changing its name to the National Foundation for Sudden Infant Death, Inc. This was done at the urging of the Roes who felt that it could no longer serve just as a memorial to Mark but should be a memorial to all victims of SIDS.

The move to New York and the change of name did not alter the fact that it was a volunteer operation. The office, equipment and telephone were donated by the Siegals; volunteers staffed the office on a rotating basis; and stationers and printers were corralled into donating their products and services. Most of the money still went directly to solving the problem. This did not last long.

The emphasis placed on public education began to take its toll on the volunteers. The lay and medical press began to write more frequently about the "mystery killer." More and more families reached the foundation's door. Materials were developed and printed with vigor. A newsletter was distributed on a regular basis, and a few dedicated volunteers spent ninety percent of their time working at establishing a true national organization. In 1968, the first full-time salaried employee was hired to function as the Executive Secretary and to direct the volunteers in the day to day operation of the foundation. The Executive Secretary was an SIDS mother and spent an increasing amount of her time dealing with other families throughout the world while the direction of the foundation remained primarily the concern of its Board of Trustees.

In the fall of 1970, the foundation again changed gears. The Executive Secretary was replaced by an Executive Administrator and new emphasis was placed on the development of a national organization with less importance attached to the grant program which had not been bringing results. An extensive evaluation was made, priorities and goals were established, greater control of the day to day activities of the foundation was placed in the hands of the one employee and the foundation began a major campaign on behalf of all SIDS victims and their families.

The campaign began with the First National Parent Medical Conference on Sudden Infant Death Syndrome held in Chicago, Illinois in July 1971. For the first time, research physicians and families from all over the United States really "heard" each other. Representatives of the federal government, the press and the medical community observed a growing force of indignation and outrage. Three days of intense discussion was the proving ground.

The "cause" was just. Families who had lost babies to the syndrome had every right to expect more than they had been getting. It sealed the bond of understanding between research physician and parent. It created a unique commitment from the newly initiated volunteer and intensified that of his long-time counterpart. Nothing new was presented, no miracle cure, just a feeling of intense caring. At long last, national attention would be focused on the problem and some significance would be given to the deaths of thousands of children.

Out of the 1971 Conference came a prospectus on the NFSID. Reproduced in part, it elucidates what the foundation set forth as major areas of present and future accomplishment:

> With limited resources and volunteer help, the Foundation has, in nine years, exceeded its highest expectations. Its mailing list has grown to approximately 10,000; it maintains a minimum of ten pieces of factual, supportive literature at all times; it has sponsored a national parent-medical conference on SIDS; it continues to add new chap-

ters; it provides speakers and material for newspaper articles to all parts of the country; it publishes a semi-annual newsletter and can document the help its volunteers have given to the victims' families.

The goals of the Foundation remain as they stood in 1962—the ultimate prevention of SIDS and the eradication of the needless guilt reactions in families stemming from ignorance about the disease. However, we can no longer solely depend on the determination and financial support of the NFSID family and volunteer. The problem is so enormous and urgent that we have resolved to both expand our own activities and solicit the support of other organizations in achieving our goals.

NO LONGER CAN WE ACCEPT . . .

1. . . . . a death certificate diagnosis, in SIDS cases, of "interstitial pneumonitis," "tracheal bronchitis," "suffocation" or any other meaningless diagnosis. Physicians must know that SIDS is a *disease*, readily diagnosed during the course of a simple autopsy. More important, parents must know that their babies have died from a specific entity.

2. . . . . callous coroners' or medical examiners' administrative procedures whereby families are kept waiting months for autopsy results or subjected to cruel inquests in SIDS cases.

3. . . . . physicians confusing all sudden, unexpected infant deaths with true SIDS. The condition can be diagnosed and must be for the sake of statistical identification and the emotional health of the family.

4. . . . . suspicion of neglect on the part of firemen, policemen, morticians, newspapermen and even clergymen with the unexpected death of an infant. These people are most often the first in contact with the stricken family; their lack of information can only further add to the feelings of guilt, grief and frustration in the family.

5. . . . . the fact that some families are denied autopsies because of lack of funds or that low income families,

not receiving private medical care, rarely receive any information about the syndrome.

6. .... the lack of instruction about SIDS in medical and other health professional schools. Without knowledge, there will be no impetus for new research nor will young physicians and nurses be prepared to deal with the syndrome should it occur in the course of their professional careers.

7. .... the existence of only a handful of research projects into the cause (or causes) of SIDS.

8. .... the lack of knowledge of the syndrome on the part of pediatricians and family physicians. Every doctor should be prepared to offer the family more than the small consolation of "these things happen."

9. .... newspaper articles of syndicated doctors' columns discussing suffocation, allergy or countless other unsubstantiated theories as the cause of SIDS. This kind of misinformation has done and continues to do, incalculable harm.

10. .... the fact that volunteer families have been asked to, alone, form local parent groups. This is a monumental undertaking which has, in the past, been directed by mail and telephone from the NFSID in New York.

WE, THEREFORE, PROPOSE ...

1. .... a standardized procedure in every community for handling cases of infants who die suddenly and unexpectedly that is both compassionate and medically sound. Autopsies must be performed and parents promptly informed of the results.

2. .... that the criteria for the diagnosis of SIDS be disseminated to coroners and medical examiners throughout the United States, and that the term, "Sudden Infant Death Syndrome," be utilized on death certificates.

3. .... that every SIDS family receive authoritative information about SIDS from a physician, nurse, or other

health professional who is both knowledgeable about the disease and skilled in dealing with characteristic grief reactions.

4. .... that a major effort be undertaken to increase the amount of research being conducted on SIDS through solicitation of the scientific community by the National Institute of Child Health and Human Development.

5. .... that parent volunteer groups be available in every state or large community to promote the aims of the Foundation on a local level. Close ties should be maintained with local physicians, particularly pediatricians and pathologists.

STRATEGY

1. Strengthening of the national office of NFSID to provide:
   a. Authoritative public information,
   b. A speaker's bureau,
   c. Consultants to assist in formation of local chapters,
   d. Liaison with other organizations.

2. Alliance with professional medical and health organizations (e.g., pediatricians, pathologists, nurses, social workers, etc.) so that they can educate their own members about SIDS.

3. Involvement of national, state and local government to:
   a. Promote SIDS research,
   b. Upgrade autopsy procedures,
   c. Disseminate authoritative information through health departments, coroner's and medical examiner's officies and law enforcement agencies by means of literature, seminars, consultants, etc.

4. A dignified public relations campaign to educate the public about SIDS without producing undue anxiety. Educational efforts will be specifically directed towards those most apt to come into contact with SIDS, such as morticians, clergy, police and firemen, and media representatives.

A PLEA

While one in every 350 live births will be a victim of
the sudden death syndrome, the National Foundation for
Sudden Infant Death, Inc. asks the assistance of all agencies and individuals concerned with the welfare of not only
the child, but the entire family unit. With the lack of
knowledge in the community, the inhumanity of most of
our autopsy systems and continuing medical misinformation, the family of the SIDS victim is shattered.

The National Foundation for Sudden Infant Death, Inc.
asks that each and every family experiencing an SIDS be
given the chance to face the death with knowledge and
dignity. We have pledged our entire resources to this end.
We request your help in making dignity a part of the lives
of 10,000 families a year.

Whatever progress has been made over the years has been
made not because the medical community saw a problem
and wanted to solve it, but because families who faced the
problem refused to believe that they couldn't at least try to
solve it. The commitment of these families has been the
mainstay of the foundation and it is what makes the parent
group unique.

The national office of the NFSID is currently staffed by
an executive director and two assistants, all salaried. But
the real work—the day to day immersion in tragedy—is
still carried on by local volunteers in their own homes.
Almost all of them belong to families who have lost babies
to the syndrome. They have refused to allow grief to im-
pede their energies, choosing instead to help others face the
crisis and to change community attitudes about SIDS. It is
no small task.

They come from all walks of life and none have been
trained for the role of counselor or political activist. Some
have substantial financial and social resources while most are
average Americans. They are families who were treated well

by their communities and families who were either mal-
treated or ignored. They usually begin their involvement
with the simple desire to help others, but for many this quiet
humanitarian act leads to intense medical and political community involvement.

Women who never expected to be anything more than
wives and mothers find themselves facing medical and legal
authorities and demanding a change in community policies.
Fathers find their garages turned into chapter headquarters.
Families learn to live with cold dinners on their tables and
frightened, grief-stricken young parents in their living rooms.

For many, the volunteer worker will be the only person
who can answer their questions, understand their grief, and
guide them through their crisis. Volunteers have been of
incalculable assistance to families who go on to have a subsequent child or who choose to adopt children. The efficiency
of the volunteers rests solely on the fact that they have been
through the same tragedy and have gone on to face their
lives in a positive manner. It is a rather sad commentary on
the delivery of health services in the United States that
unless SIDS families in a community organize to help others
like themselves, that community will be without services.

Until a nationwide procedure for the handling of sudden unexpected infant deaths is developed, the NFSID will
maintain the establishment of local chapters as a high priority. The community services offered by a chapter are
scaled to reach the stricken family, the general public and
those members of the community whose professions would
indicate contact with a family (i.e., pediatricians, funeral
directors, clergy, etc.). The programs are set to reach all
families in the community so that they may know immediately why their baby died and to whom they can turn for
information and aid.

The early growth of the foundation was sustained by the

financial commitment of the Roes and their associates. The continued growth has been supported, on the whole, by memorial contributions and the financial sacrifices of all the volunteers. Although recent years have seen a small increase in grants and outside foundation support, funds have not been easily obtained. Life-sustaining machinery and hospital wings carrying name plates are far more inviting then public education campaigns, development of health services and the production of authoritative materials.

However, the National Foundation for Sudden Infant Death, Inc. continues to increase its financial commitment to research, education, and the development of a humane system of handling Sudden Infant Death Syndrome. An increasing amount of time is spent on fund-raising activities and solicitations to support that commitment. We are certain that this is true of the other organizations concerned with the same problem. If no one else comes through, families will continue to make personal sacrifices and support the goals of the foundation. As long as there is *one* parent left who feels responsible for their child's death, all families will unite in parent groups to tell them that they are NOT.

VIII

POLITICS AND SIDS

"What with all the job changes over there, the busiest people in this town must be the sign painters down at the Department of Health, Education and Welfare."

Senator Warren G. Magnuson (D-Wash.)

Dr. Abraham Bergman has been accused, from time to time (though he doesn't necessarily view it as an accusation) of being a political activist who happens to be a physician. That characterization is not too far off the mark. He believes politicians have the capacity to save many more lives than physicians. (The converse is also true. They can also sacrifice more lives than physicians.)

One day in 1966, he had lunch with a high school classmate, an attorney, who was working for the Senate Commerce Committee. Dr. Bergman complained about the menace of rotary lawn mowers; he'd seen children at the hospital severely injured by machines which lacked the most elementary safety devices. His friend said, "If you're really worried about the problem, why don't you do something about it instead of writing just another article for a journal that's only read by doctors?" The friend was right, of course. Physicians expend a great deal of energy and time talking only to each other.

Dr. Bergman gave his friend a copy of a paper he'd written for a medical journal on the subject, and his friend promptly showed it to *his* boss, Senator Warren G. Magnuson. To Dr. Bergman's delight, within days Senator Magnuson had warned the mower industry he would attempt to pass regulatory legislation unless the industry voluntarily adopted an adequate safety code. They didn't and he did! A law was passed establishing the Consumer Product Safety Commission with the power to regulate the safety of all household products, including power lawn mowers.

Dr. Bergman found that there *is* a way to effect some degree of change in health care by dealing directly with those responsible for the passage of the necessary legislation. Senator Magnuson, the senior senator from the state of Washington, is enormously interested in health care problems. As Chairman of the United States Senate's Labor HEW Appropriations subcommittee which is responsible for appropriations for the Department of Health, Education and Welfare, he is in a position to influence the passage of health care legislation. At Bergman's instigation, he has sponsored several critical health measures, most notably the Flammable Fabrics Act, Poison Prevention Act and the National Health Service Corps. The Magnuson subcommittee is responsible for HEW funding and in turn for appropriations for the National Institute of Child Health and Human Development (NICHHD). The senator and his staff assistants, particularly Harley M. Dirks, Magnuson's chief aide on the Appropriations subcommittee, have kept up pressure on the administration to commit more funds for SIDS research.

From its inception, NICHHD has given high priority to the problem of Sudden Infant Death Syndrome. Through its first two directors, the institute has had a close association with the University of Washington. When NICHHD was created in 1963, as part of the Department of Health, Education and Welfare, President Kennedy appointed the

Chairman of the Department of Pediatrics at the University of Washington, Dr. Robert Aldrich, as the first director. Aldrich, who is presently Vice President for Health Affairs at the University of Colorado, was sensitized to the SIDS problem by the Dores and other Seattle parents. When Aldrich assumed his position at NICHHD, he brought with him from Seattle as the head of the Mental Retardation Division, Dr. Gerald LaVeck. Dr. LaVeck had trained at the University of Washington, served with the Public Health Service as Director of the Rainier School (for the mentally retarded) near Seattle, and as Director of the Crippled Children's Services of the Washington State Health Department. When Dr. Aldrich left NICHHD in 1966, LaVeck took over as the Institute's second director.

The interest in SIDS at the Child Health Institute was sustained because of the encouragement of these two directors. Encouragement was about the only thing they had to offer, however, because funds for SIDS research were scant and the trained scientists willing to work on the problem even more scarce. In terms of the overall priorities of the National Institutes of Health, SIDS could not be found even in the small print.

A special vote of thanks must be extended to one individual at NICHHD who, through the 1960's, patiently promoted research in SIDS. He is Dr. Dwain Walcher, a virologist who for some time was the Institute's Associate Director for Program Planning and Evaluation. Dr. Walcher served as the "godfather" to investigators of SIDS and set a high standard as both a dedicated scientist and public servant.

When Dr. Walcher left NICHHD in 1969, responsibility for shepherding the SIDS research program was given to Dr. Eileen Hasselmayer, who holds a doctorate in nursing, and Mr. Jehu Hunter, a scientist-administrator with a background in biochemistry. They didn't have much to work with. During the fiscal year of 1971, the federal government funded only a single grant specifically directed to the cause of SIDS at a level of $46,258 (the Seattle study, directed then by Dr. Ray).

THE MONDALE HEARINGS

If 1963 marks the time when SIDS research became "respectable" in scientific circles, 1972 marks the year when the public became conscious of this mysterious and tragic disease. The form was a hearing before the Senate's Subcommittee on Children and Youth chaired by Senator Walter Mondale (Democrat-Minnesota). The Mondale subcommittee had been looking at a series of problems affecting children in the United States and was responsible for important legislation concerning day-care facilities for children from disadvantaged families.

Frustrated by the lack of attention being given to SIDS research by the National Institutes of Health, SIDS parents had bombarded their congressmen with letters of protest. The letter-writing campaign was spearheaded by members of the Guild for Infant Survival which is centered in Baltimore. Senator Mondale and his colleagues decided to act, and in so doing set the stage for one of the most dramatic hearings held on Capitol Hill in many years. Three networks showed up on January 25, 1972 to televise the hearing, an act which always heightens interest among politicians. Although there were official witnesses representing the administration, the American Academy of Pediatrics, and the National Foundation for Sudden Infant Death, the most dramatic testimony came from parents themselves. Frank Hennigan, a prominent business executive in Chicago, gave the briefest but most moving testimony as he related how he was harrassed by law enforcement officers and the press after his baby died of SIDS. Excerpts from the hearing appeared on television and in newspapers throughout the country. The NFSID was invited to the TODAY show, which in turn led to many appearances on local television channels.

As a result of the hearings, Senator Mondale and fifteen co-sponsors introduced Senate Joint Resolution 206, relating to Sudden Infant Death Syndrome. The text of the resolution reads as follows:

Joint Resolution
Relating to sudden infant death syndrome.

Whereas sudden infant death syndrome kills more infants between the age of one month and one year than any other disease; and

Whereas the cause and prevention of sudden infant death syndrome are unknown; and

Whereas there is a lack of adequate knowledge about the disease and its effects among the public and professionals who come into contact with it; Therefore be it

Resolved by the Senate and House of Representatives of the United States of America in Congress assembled, That it is the purpose of this joint resolution to assure that the maximum resources and effort be concentrated on medical research into sudden infant death syndrome and on the extension of services to families who lose children to the disease.

SEC. 2. The National Institute of Child Health and Human Development, of the Department of Health, Education, and Welfare, is hereby directed to designate the search for a cause and prevention of sudden infant death syndrome as one of the top priorities in intramural research efforts and in the awarding of research and research training grants and fellowships; and to encourage researchers to submit proposals for investigations of sudden infant death syndrome.

SEC. 3. The Secretary of Health, Education, and Welfare is directed to develop, publish and distribute literature to be used in educating and counseling coroners, medical examiners, nurses, social workers, and similar personnel and parents, future parents, and families whose children die, to the nature of sudden infant death syndrome and to the needs of families affected by it.

SEC. 4. The Secretary of Health, Education, and Welfare is further directed to work toward the institution of statistical reporting procedures that will provide a reliable index to the incidence and distribution of sudden infant death syndrome cases throughout the Nation; to work toward the availability of autopsies of children who apparently die of sudden infant death syndrome and for prompt release of the results to their parents; and to add sudden infant death syndrome to the International Classification of Disease.

The resolution was reported out of the Committee and sent to the Senate floor, passing by a vote of seventy-seven to zero.

The Senate also acted to increase the appropriation for SIDS research. President Nixon had requested no funds in the National Institutes of Health specifically for SIDS research. Led by Senator Magnuson, the Senate provided ten million dollars for specific SIDS research. It was later halved to four million dollars after a conference with the House. Calling it inflationary, the President vetoed the HEW appropriation bill in 1971 and again in 1972. Certainly SIDS research was not the point of issue—there were much bigger increases to which the President objected—but the fact remains that a major expansion in SIDS research was hindered by the confrontation between President Nixon and Congress over who should set priorities on government spending.

The attention given to SIDS in Congress during 1971 and the desire of powerful senators and representatives for action was not lost upon the directors of the National Institutes of Health. Even though NICHHD did not receive extra money specifically earmarked for SIDS, the institute allocated money from other programs to expand the research effort in SIDS. They did what should have been done ten years ago—went out and actively solicited research proposals from scientists who previously knew little if anything about the problem. Advertisements were taken in major scientific journals alerting scientists to the availability of research funds for SIDS, an attractive lure at a time when most research grants were being cut back. Two important projects were finally funded: the studies of Dr. Alfred Steinschneider of Syracuse on the development of breathing patterns in young babies; and a study on the mechanisms of sleep in young infants, began by Dr. Maurice Sterman, a noted researcher in the field of sleep physiology at the Veteran's Administration Hospital at Sepulveda, California, in cooperation with Dr. Joan Hodgman at the Los Angeles County Hospital.

While the research arm of HEW was active, the rest of the department lay inert when it came to dealing with the SIDS problem. The Maternal and Child Health Service, which has recently been reorganized out of existence, did provide thirty thousand dollars to produce an educational movie on SIDS and five thousand dollars to launch regional educational seminars. But only after Senator Magnuson asked his aide Mr. Dirks to make a few phone calls.

Twenty months after the first Mondale Hearings, a joint hearing before Mondale's Subcommittee on Children and Youth and Senator Kennedy's Subcommittee on Health was held in Washington on September 20, 1973. The joint hearing was held for the purpose of hearing testimony on behalf of S 1745; a bill to "provide financial assistance for research activities for the study of Sudden Infant Death Syndrome, to provide *information* and *counseling* services to families. . . ." S 1745 further proposed the establishment of regional medical centers for the study of the disease, a proposal which one of the authors (Bergman) had recommended for over a year.

Again the attention of the nation was focused on the plight of parents of SIDS victims. Moving testimony was offered by John and Patricia Smiley of California who'd been charged, jailed and later released—all in connection with the sudden death of their baby. This is a dramatic example of the need for federal action that was further enforced by strong supportive testimony by nationally recognized medicolegal authorities.

After some months of conference committee deliberations between the Senate and the House of Representatives, The Sudden Infant Death Syndrome Act of 1974 was made Public Law 93-270 with President Richard M. Nixon's signature on April 23, 1974. The text of this landmark legislation follows:

SHORT TITLE

SECTION 1. This Act may be cited as the "Sudden Infant Death Syndrome Act of 1974."

SUDDEN INFANT DEATH SYNDROME RESEARCH

SEC. 2. (a) Section 441 of the Public Health Service Act is amended by striking out "an institute" and inserting in lieu thereof "the National Institute of Child Health and Human Development."

(b) (1) Such section 441 is further amended by inserting "(a)" after "Sec. 441." and by adding at the end thereof the following:

"(b) The Secretary shall carry out through the National Institute of Child Health and Human Development the purposes of section 301 with respect to the conduct and support of research which specifically relates to sudden infant death syndrome."

(2) Section 444 of such Act is amended (1) by striking out "The Surgeon General" each place it occurs and inserting in lieu thereof "The Secretary," and (2) by striking out "the Surgeon General shall, with the approval of the Secretary" in the first sentence and inserting in lieu thereof "the Secretary shall, in accordance with section 441(b),".

(c) (1) Within 90 days following the close of the fiscal year ending June 30, 1975, and the close of each of the next two fiscal years, the Secretary shall report to the Committees on Appropriations of the Senate and the House of Representatives and to the Committee on Labor and Public Welfare of the Senate and the Committee on Interstate and Foreign Commerce of the House of Representatives the following information for such fiscal year:

(A) The (i) number of applications approved by the Secretary in the fiscal year reported on for grants and contracts under the Public Health Service Act for research which relates specifically to sudden infant death syndrome, (ii) total amount requested under such applications, (iii) number of such applications for which funds were provided in such fiscal year, and (iv) total amount of such funds.

(B) The (i) number of applications approved by the Secretary in such fiscal year for grants and contracts under the Public Health Service Act for research which relates generally to sudden infant death syndrome, (ii) total amount requested under such applications, (iii) number of such applications for which funds were provided in such fiscal year, and (iv) total amount of such funds.

Each such report shall contain an estimate of the need for additional funds for grants or contracts under the Public Health Service Act for research which relates specifically to sudden infant death syndrome.

(2) Within five days after the Budget is transmitted by the President to the Congress for the fiscal year ending June 30, 1976, and for each of the next two fiscal years, the Secretary shall transmit to the Committee on Appropriations of the House of Representatives and the Senate, the Committee on Labor and Public Welfare of the Senate, and the Committees on Interstate and Foreign Commerce of the House of Representatives an estimate of the amount requested for the National Institutes of Health for research to sudden infant death syndrome and a comparison of that amount with

the amount requested for the preceding fiscal year.

COUNSELING, INFORMATION, EDUCATIONAL AND STATISTICAL PROGRAMS

SEC. 3. (a) Title XI of the Public Health Service Act is amended by adding at the end thereof the following new part:

PART C—SUDDEN INFANT DEATH SYNDROME

"SUDDEN INFANT DEATH SYNDROME COUNSELING, INFORMATION, EDUCATIONAL, AND STATISTICAL PROGRAMS

"SEC. 1121. (a) The Secretary, through the Assistant Secretary for Health, shall carry out a program to develop public information and professional educational materials relating to sudden infant death syndrome and to disseminate such information and materials to persons providing health care, to public safety officials, and to the public generally.

"(b) (1) The Secretary may make grants to public and nonprofit private entities and enter into contracts with public and private entities, for projects which include both—

"(A) the collection, analysis, and furnishing of information (derived from post mortem examinations and other means) relating to the causes of sudden infant death syndrome; and

"(B) the provision of information and counseling to families affected by sudden infant death syndrome.

"(2) No grant may be made or contract entered into under this subsection unless an application therefor has been submitted to and approved by the Secretary. Such application shall be in such form, submitted in such manner, and contain such information as the Secretary shall be regulation prescribe. Each applicant shall—

"(A) provide that the project for which assistance under this subsection is sought will be administered by or under supervision of the applicant;

"(B) provide for appropriate community representation in the development and operation of such project;

"(C) set forth such fiscal controls and fund accounting procedures as may be necessary to assure proper disbursement of and accounting for Federal funds paid to the applicant under this subsection; and

"(D) provide for making such reports in such form and containing such information as the Secretary may reasonably require.

"(3) Payments under grants under this subsection may be in advance or by way of reimbursement, and at such intervals and on such conditions, as the Secretary finds necessary.

"(4) Contracts under this subsection may be entered into without regard to sections 3648 through 3709 of the Revised Statutes (31 U.S.C. 529; 44 U.S.C. 5).

"(5) For the purpose of making payments pursuant to grants and contracts under this subsection, there are authorized to be appropriated $2,000,000 for the fiscal year ending June 30, 1975, $3,000,000 for the fiscal year ending June 30, 1976, and $4,000,000 for the fiscal year ending June 30, 1977.

"(c) The Secretary shall submit, not later than January 1, 1976, a comprehensive report to the Committee on Labor and Public Welfare of the Senate and the Committee on Interstate and Foreign Commerce of the House of Representatives respecting the administration of this section and the results obtained from the programs authorized by it."

(b) The title of such title XI is amended by adding at the end thereof "AND SUDDEN INFANT DEATH SYNDROME."

The motion was agreed to.

Public Law 93-270 has only lately been funded and its fate is not yet known. What is important, however, is that SIDS has moved, with authority, into the political arena.

While HEW and the National Institute of Child Health have allocated funds for research into the causes of SIDS, there is enormous inertia in those agencies regarding the more "human" aspects of SIDS. Dr. Bergman has been to see officials at HEW countless times about applying themselves to this side of the problem. Every official he's spoken with at HEW has promised to "do something" and yet we wait and wait and wait.

Government officials in Washington are always very busy with *big problems*. SIDS, the leading killer of children under a year of age carries a very low priority. No sense of urgency exists. There are plenty of difficult problems in this country for which solutions are *not* available. The problems of thousands of SIDS parents feeling responsible for killing their children is, of course, not one of the larger problems of our society ... BUT IT IS SO EMINENTLY SOLVABLE.

IX

THE CURRENT MANAGEMENT OF THE SUDDEN INFANT DEATH SYNDROME IN THE UNITED STATES

". . . it does seem remarkable that everyone can concede that this major cause of deaths is a particularly mysterious and hideous form of death and yet the best minds of American medicine are largely taking public opinion polls at this time on the matter."

Senator Walter F. Mondale (D.-Minn.)
January 25, 1972
United States Senate Subcommittee
on Children and Youth

During the summer of 1972, the Children's Orthopedic Hospital and Medical Center and the University of Washington School of Public Health and Community Medicine in Seattle undertook a nation wide study of the management of SIDS, under the sponsorship of the National Institute of Child Health and Human Development. Ten teams of two graduate students each visited 148 counties in 48 states (Hawaii and Alaska were excluded). Information was obtained from 145 coroners and medical examiners, 421 parents, plus a variety of other physicians and public officials.

It should be stressed that the picture presented below was obtained in 1972. Fortunately, many improvements took place subsequent to the study. Only 27% of the officials certi· fying the cause of death were pathologists; 30% were physicians other than pathologists; 9% were morticians; 4% justices of the peace; 3% lawyers, and 27% were laymen with no medical or legal qualifications.

In general, across the country, the autopsy rate correlated with the funds available. Small counties without a salaried pathologist usually have a definite sum of money set aside for securing autopsies from private pathologists. There is great reluctance to use these funds for crib death (SIDS) cases, which are assumed to be natural deaths. Rather, the funds are generally used to investigate deaths in which foul play is suspected. Only in 25% of the communities studied were autopsies performed on all sudden unexplained deaths. In 20% of the communities, the policy was that autopsies were not to be performed unless the official had a definite suspicion of an unlawful act. In the remaining communities, the performance of an autopsy depended primarily on the personal inclination of the coroner or medical examiner, available funds, and on whether a private physician or family insisted on it. Even in such large communities as Boston and Chicago, both with world famous medical centers, less than a third of crib death cases are autopsied.

Coroner and medical examiner log books for the three-year period 1969–71 were examined by the study teams. An incredible variety of terminology was used to describe crib death. Among them were: Sudden Infant Death Syndrome, sudden unexpected infant death, sudden death in infancy, pneumonia, interstitial pneumonitis, respiratory infection, acute necrotizing laryngitis, crib suffocation, anoxia due to undetermined cause, aspiration of vomitus, suffocation under bedclothes, acute tracheobronchitis and pulmonary edema.

Some coroners associate crib death with child abuse or neglect. For example, the Ada County (Idaho) coroner saw the cause of crib death as "partial neglect and quick pneumonia." The coroner of Jefferson County (Alabama) thought that many crib deaths are due to suffocation because "blacks do not know how to care for their children properly." He cited as evidence the practice of children sleeping in the same bed as their parents, which he felt led to death by suffocation.

Parents who lose infants to SIDS often wait in agonizing suspense to hear the results of the autopsy. In two thirds of the communities studied where autopsies are performed, families had to wait weeks, even months, to learn the cause of their children's deaths.

Considerable discrepancy was noted between the information provided by officials and that provided by the parents with respect to notification of cause of death. Sixty percent (60%) of coroners or medical examiners responded that they routinely notify parents of the cause of death, usually by telephone. The converse is that 40% of officials have *no* established notification procedure. Even in the areas where the officials said their office routinely notifies the families, it is the families who initiate the contact before they get any word.

We consider the question of whether or not a family had to initiate contact with the coroner or medical examiner to receive the results of the autopsy as a crucial point in the management process. It is obvious to us that the poorer families were less verbal, less apt to have telephones, and generally tend to be less bold in dealing with such establishment institutions as the coroner or medical examiner's office. The social class difference did indeed count in this category: 41% of lower-class families had to initiate contact as compared to 29% of middle-class and 34% of upper-class families.

Families in lower income brackets, where SIDS incidence is higher, usually do not have private physicians and tend to be neglected if not dismissed. When a family had a knowledgeable private physician, it stood a better chance of receiving proper information and not suffering unnecessary guilt reactions.

From the parents interviewed, we learned that police or fire personnel were the most likely officials on the scene after the infant was discovered lifeless. There were some abuses such as the parents who were jailed, but on the whole families praised the efforts of policemen and firemen who responded to their calls for help. On the other hand, a great deal of resentment was expressed towards hospital emergency room personnel (physicians and nurses) who were indifferent and sometimes accusatory. Only half the families were told that the deaths were caused by SIDS, crib death or similar terminology. The others were given explanations like pneumonia or suffocation. Ten percent (10%) of the families interviewed never received any explanation as to why their babies died. Eighty three percent (83%) said that the verbal explanation given them at the time of the death was not the same as what was later listed on the death certificate. Only 49% of the families felt that the cause of death was adequately explained to them by anyone.

Parent groups, either the NFSID (National Foundation for Sudden Infant Death) or GIS (Guild for Infant Survival), were felt to be extremely helpful by families who came in contact with them. The majority of the communities studied, however, did not have active parent groups and even in those that did, the organizations simply didn't reach lower socio-economic class families. For example, the parent group was considered to be *the* most helpful person or organization by 25 of the 293 (9%) of upper and middle-class families. *None* of the 75 lower-class families included in the study mentioned a member of a parent group as being the most helpful person to them.

An abstract from the final report prepared on the study follows.

Abstract of Study Report
The Management of Sudden Infant Death Syndrome (SIDS) in the United States (1972)

How do stricken families, physicians, coroners, medical examiners, pathologists, policemen, firemen, nurses, neighbors, relatives and friends react to the always unexpected and still unpredictable event of a sudden infant death—commonly called a crib death?

What is the outcome of false, ignorant, and sometimes callous reactions to the tragedy now properly and precisely described as the Sudden Infant Death Syndrome (acronym SIDS)—exact cause unknown, prevention still impossible, outcome uniformly fatal?

Documented and useful answers to these and allied questions are to be found in this nationwide study of 421 families in which SIDS had occurred and of the professional personnel (e.g., physicians, medical examiners) concerned with these deaths. The interviews were conducted in the summer of 1972.

The regular sequence of events in SIDS is commonly this: An apparently healthy infant, usually between the ages of two weeks and four months, is put to sleep for the night in his crib. The next morning, or even earlier, the infant is discovered dead in the crib. No outcry has been heard.

Emergency services are summoned—police, firemen, physicians, ambulances. The infant is usually rushed to a local hospital and pronounced dead on arrival.

The parents are stunned, grief-stricken; they usually have no idea what has happened. Too often they are not made aware of what has occurred; sometimes they are opening or subtly *accused* of having caused their child's death.

According to this study, 14% of the afflicted parents *never* learn why their infants died. Fifty percent (50%) feel they were not given an adequate explanation. In about one third (33%) of the cases, the parents are *told* one cause of death and *see* another cause written on the infant's death certificate.

In order to ascertain the cause of any sudden infant death (causes other than SIDS may be properly assigned in about 15% of the cases) an autopsy is essential. Only in half the communities covered in the present study were autopsies routinely performed. Big cities like Boston and Chicago had an autopsy rate of less than 30%.

Marked racial and social class distinctions were found to exist in the professional and official handling of SIDS parents. Families without private physicians tended to receive the worst care and the least attention. But relatively few families, rich or poor, had any idea about SIDS until it struck their own home. The higher the educational level of the family, the more likely they were to have known about SIDS before it hit.

In too many families, for reasons already outlined, the outcome of SIDS is a profound and often prolonged grief and guilt reaction. While SIDS itself is not now predictable or preventable, the psychiatric casualties trailing after it can be prevented or largely eased by proper, professional, and kindly management of the members of the family wherein SIDS has occurred.

The shortcomings uncovered by this study could be overcome by the establishment of regional centers serving a defined geographic area where all cases of sudden, unexpected death would be autopsied with families receiving appropriate information and counseling.

RATIONALE OF STUDY

Much confusion and much ignorance about SIDS currently prevails both in the health professions and among the lay public. Sudden infant deaths are handled in a variety of ways throughout the country, particularly with respect to autopsy procedures, death certificate terminology, and information given to families.

A standardized method of managing sudden infant death cases throughout the country might alleviate some of the psychiatric morbidity that so frequently erupts among surviving family members. But before case-management standards can be recommended, it is essential to obtain an accurate picture of current practices with respect to SIDS throughout the entire country.

In essence, this study was undertaken to determine, at least in the continental United States:

1. How SIDS cases are actually handled by physicians, coroners, medical examiners and other professionals
2. Where "good" management and "bad" management of SIDS cases prevail, this being the thrust of Part II, Summary of Observations by Locality
3. What significant effects on SIDS families may result from good, not so good, and even bad management of the misfortune that has struck them.

DISCUSSION AND RECOMMENDATIONS

As stated in the preface, this study assumes that a minimum acceptable standard of handling Sudden Infant Death Syndrome should exist in all communities throughout the United States. The elements of this standard are:

1. Autopsies should be available to all children who die suddenly and unexpectedly and should be performed by qualified pathologists.
2. The term "Sudden Infant Death Syndrome" should be utilized as a cause of death on death certificates.
3. Families should be notified of the autopsy results within 24 hours.
4. Follow-up information about SIDS and counseling should be provided by a knowledgeable health professional.

These standards have also been advocated by the American Academy of Pediatrics.

The study showed that in the summer of 1972 the level of service outlined above was available in only a handful of American communities. Smaller counties are hard put to investigate obvious criminal cases, let alone cope adequately with natural disease problems such as Sudden Infant Death Syndrome. It is unrealistic for a small community with no pathologist, small funds, and inadequate facilities to do post-mortems on all babies.

RECOMMENDATIONS

SIDS victims should be transported to designated *regional centers* staffed by competent pathologists. Such regional centers would be best suited to deal with the unique problem of SIDS. In some area, the centers could be situated with the medical examiner office or coroner office where there are already existing resources. In other areas, a university medical center or affiliated teaching hospital would be the most appropriate places. The decision as to which alternative would best serve the community and region should be a local one. Regional and state comprehensive health-planning agencies should assist in determining the appropriate location of these centers.

AUTOPSIES

Enabling state legislation *might* be necessary in some states to allow the transport of SIDS victims across county lines and to allow autopsies to be performed outside of coroner or medical examiner offices. Such laws exist in the states of Washington and Oregon.

Because of the medical examiners' and coroners' legal responsibilities, it is necessary that they still maintain a connection with the case even if the post-mortem is performed outside their local jurisdiction. Cases involving criminal action must still be referred to these officials. It is often helpful if the pathologist performing the autopsy is appointed as a deputy medical examiner or coroner.

Consideration should be given to providing federal matching funds for the establishment and maintenance of such regional centers with state and county government, as well as other sources, sharing the cost. The condition for receipt of federal matching funds should be performance of the minimum services outlined above.

DIAGNOSIS OF SIDS

Extreme variability exists among pathologists about the diagnosis of SIDS. The following statement, expressing his own personal philosophy about the diagnosis of SIDS, has been prepared by J. Bruce Beckwith, M.D., pathologist at Children's Orthopedic Hospital and Medical Center in Seattle. Though it is unrealistic to expect that all pathologists will agree with all parts of the statement, adoption of its principles would clearly be a more effective means of "humanizing" the handling of SIDS. It is, thus, included as a recommendation in this report.

RECOMMENDATION:

I. The diagnosis of SIDS at autopsy involves two issues—scientific and humanistic. It is necessary that one be willing to render a reasonably positive diagnosis immediately if effective counseling is to be accomplished. We, therefore, make a diagnosis of SIDS *for counseling purposes* on the basis of gross autopsy findings alone in the vast majority of instances. If subsequent workup reveals additional information, and we deem this important for the family to know, we so notify them. Usually our approach is to tell them the infant did in fact die of SIDS, but in working up the case in detail, something was found which we feel they should know about. Usually this pertains if an unsuspected genetically determined condition is found.

II. I have just reviewed 500 consecutive carefully studied sudden unexpected deaths in infants and children aged one day to three years in the Seattle study. Of these, 425 or *85 percent* were diagnosed as SIDS. This should give an approximate baseline against which these series can be measured. If significantly larger or smaller percentages of unexpected infant deaths are being termed SIDS, then criteria for the diagnosis should be reviewed.

III. Of infants in the above study who were (1) under one year of age, (2) apparently died during a sleeping period, and (3) showed no obvious external signs of lethal disease, then 92 *percent* were eventually diagnosed as SIDS.

IV. The diagnosis of SIDS is made on two bases, exclusional and inclusional. The former is by far the more important. We rule out gross starvation or dehydration by external examination, supplemented by thymic weight. A significantly atrophic thymus should cause suspicion of an underlying stressful condition. Meningitis or head injury is ruled out by examination of the brain grossly. Obvious enteric or renal disease sufficient to cause death is also easily diagnosed. The larynx should be examined to rule out epiglottitic and aspirated objects. The criteria we use with respect to the *respiratory system* are as follows:

1. Bronchopneumonia rather than SIDS is diagnosed when there is *grossly obvious, purulent consolidation* (as opposed to the uniform somewhat firm, rubbery texture of congested, edematous lungs usually seen in SIDS). Usually this consolidation is localized to some degree, and offers a striking contrast to adjacent more normal lung. Fibrin or pus is found on the overlying pleura. If the microscope is required to diagnose pneumonia, we do not view it as an adequate cause for death.

2. Tracheobronchitis is diagnosed when the trachea or major bronchi are *occluded by pus*. This is not to be confused with flecks of milk, or frothy edema fluid.

V. *SIDS typically shows congested, edematous lungs*

and intrathoracic petechiae. *We see these in over 85% of cases, but do not demand their presence to make the diagnosis.*

VI. Typical SIDS cases die during apparent sleep, and are under one year of age. There are no alarming symptoms and no externally obvious lethal abnormalities. Any case that is over one year, was observed to die, or otherwise differs from the above, is probably not SIDS, but sometimes nothing else is found, and the diagnosis can then be made at least for counseling purposes.

VII. Operationally, I certify deaths as follows, *at the time of gross autopsy*:

1. (Typical SIDS history, no gross cause of death) —"SIDS is certified."

2. (Atypical case by virtue of history, anatomically also not typical, but no gross cause of death): "No gross anatomical cause of death—studies pending."

This latter format is used for fewer than 5% of cases, especially where a real possibility of myocarditis, encephalitis, or poisoning is suspected on the basis of gross findings.

TERMINOLOGY

Not until the Second International Conference was the term Sudden Infant Death Syndrome (SIDS) formally proposed. It was rapidly utilized in medical literature and has gained almost universal acceptance among pediatricians. There is always a "lag time" for current medical knowledge to be universally applied.

An incredible variety of terminology is used by coroners and medical examiners to explain certified cases of sudden unexpected infant death. This state of confusion leaves only the parents of the SIDS victims to suffer wondering what to believe caused their child's death. It was extremely common for parents to be told one cause of death by the coroner and another cause by their private physician. The most invidious terms—suffocation, aspiration, and asphyxiation— unfortunately, are still in common use. When such terms as pneumonia or upper respiratory infection are used, parents still suffer profound guilt, blaming themselves for allowing their child to remain ill without medical attention. To lay persons, pneumonia is a disease requiring medical attention; qualifying words such as interstitial, hemorrhagic or viral, do not make the matter any better.

RECOMMENDATIONS:

A concerted educational campaign must be directed to those certifying and recording causes of death to use the term Sudden Infant Death Syndrome. Because of the tremendous harm done to parents by use of inappropriate terminology, a directive should promptly be issued by the National Center for Health Statistics (Department of H.E.W.) to all Vital Statistic Registrars to utilize the term SIDS whenever appropriate on death certificates. This *must not* be delayed for years until there is revision of the international nomenclature. State and local registrars do not all yet use the term Sudden Infant Death Syndrome or its acronym, SIDS, but they should no longer have any excuse for disregarding it when it is applicable. The effectiveness of such a directive has been demonstrated in California (November, 1971) and in Iowa (March, 1972) where the health departments issued such an order and there was an immediate and significant increase in the use of the term or acronym, SIDS, as a final diagnosis.

NOTIFICATION OF FAMILY

The notification system for informing parents of the cause of their child's death is extremely haphazard. Again, only a handful of communities have a standardized notification procedure; the vast majority of communities leave it to the parent to take the initiative in obtaining information from the coroner or medical examiner. All too many parents wait for many months or are never notified of the results of the autopsy. It is both unrealistic and inhumane to place the responsibility on shocked and grieving parents to call a coroner or medical examiner office for information. Lower social class and racial minority families really need help. They are feeling guilty anyhow, which combined with a tendency to be distrustful of public officials, profoundly inhibits them from taking the initiative to seek out information.

Routine notification of parents as soon as possible after death appeared to be extremely helpful to them in dealing with their feelings of guilt. Letters from the medical examiner or coroner explaining the cause of death were treasured by parents who received them. A few pathologists, such as J. Bruce Beckwith, M.D. of Seattle, call the family immediately after the autopsy; but this is an extremely delicate and taxing assignment and is not advocated unless the pathologist is particularly adept in communication skills.

RECOMMENDATION:

A brief letter from an official certifying the cause of death should be sent to the family immediately upon conclusion of the gross autopsy examination. (Sample letters are included in appendices to Community Profiles.) The letter should be accompanied by a printed fact sheet about SIDS. An authoritative document in their hands does much to "certify" their own blamelessness to parents as well as to relatives and friends who desire explanations.

RACIAL AND SOCIAL CLASS DIFFERENCES

Marked racial and social class discrimination in the handling of parents by officials was found in this study. Many officials felt that low income and minority families do not care for their children as well as other groups. Suspicion of neglect or abuse was foremost in their minds when called to a case of sudden unexpected death; the hostile and accusatory acts of these officials towards poor and minority families reflected their theories of child abuse. Such discriminatory practices, though existent, were not limited to the South. Blacks and Mexican-Americans tended to suffer greatly in areas where the coroner or medical examiner did not recognize SIDS as a disease entity and failed to explain the cause of the infant's death. If a family had a private physician and that physician was knowledgeable about SIDS, they were apt to be treated well and to adjust to the loss of their child. If not, they tended to be treated badly and to suffer prolonged guilt reactions unless the local coroner or medical examiner was particularly sensitive to the "human" aspects of SIDS.

RECOMMENDATION:

Public health nurses should be employed to provide information and counseling to SIDS stricken families on an organized basis. Nurses should be properly instructed and provided with special training to perform this function as it requires special skills. In Seattle and New Orleans where such a program was functioning at the time of the study, the nurses were found to carry this counseling role in a superb manner. Such a nurse should be part of a regional center working closely with the pathologist who performs the autopsy. Consistency in terms of information given to families must be maintained. The public health nurse supplements the role of a family physician and her services should not be restricted only to families who do not have their own physicians.

PSYCHIATRIC MORBIDITY

Though this study was not intended to assay the prevalence of psychiatric morbidity due to SIDS, it was apparent that mental health problems in families of crib death victims were both common and long lasting. Furthermore, other than a few SIDS parent groups, the problem is totally unrecognized and no helping services are being provided.

RECOMMENDATION:

Support for case finding should be considered to assist in referral of "abused parents" to mental health services. Concomitantly, mental health workers must be educated about the emotional aspects of SIDS. Psychiatric morbidity from SIDS will be reduced (but not eliminated) in future years, as "preventive psychiatry" in the form of humane handling of SIDS cases becomes more widespread.

PROFESSIONAL EDUCATION

At the time of the field investigation, only two local health departments and no state health departments were involved with the problem of sudden infant death. Local officials varied as to their knowledge of and interest in the problem. Only one state medical association (Washington) had any organized activity involving SIDS; county medical societies were totally uninvolved. Medical schools and teaching hospitals were, likewise, insulated from the problem.

Sadly, increasing publicity being given to another neglected problem, child abuse, has tended to direct more suspicion to families of SIDS victims. Though rare, families whose children die of SIDS are still being jailed for suspected child abuse.

RECOMMENDATION:

The Department of Health, Education and Welfare should support a nationwide effort to establish an effective educational program directed towards those who come in contact with SIDS families: physicians, nurses, social workers, firemen, morticians and clergymen. Presently, only the biomedical research aspects of SIDS are being dealt with adequately in HEW through the National Institute of Child Health and Human Development.

The Maternal and Child Health Service has sponsored a series of regional seminars and produced an educational film on SIDS subsequent to the completion of this field study. This type of activity should be significantly expanded and involve other HEW programs which could contribute, such as the National Institute of Mental Health and the National Center for Health Statistics. Strong efforts must also be made to involve state and local health departments in the problem.

PARENT ORGANIZATIONS

It is doubtful that any activity in SIDS, either in research or services to families, would have occurred without the strong efforts of the lay parent organizations, such as the National Foundation for Sudden Infant Death (NFSID) and the Guild for Infant Survival (GIS). The communities which have set up humane programs for handling SIDS families have done so only because of the combination of a strong parent group and a responsive coroner or medical examiner. Interestingly, as the lay organizations grow, more individuals who are not SIDS parents are beginning to play active roles. Up to now, parents who have lost children to SIDS have had to bear the brunt of counseling newly bereaved families, mostly because there was no one else available to do the job. Both the NFSID and GIS consist primarily of white middle-class families; neither organization has been successful in reaching low income and minority families. Such families do not tend to be "joiners." Thus, reliance should not be placed on the lay organizations to provide counseling services to SIDS families. That is a delicate task that should be done by individuals, such as nurses or social workers, with some training in dealing with grief reactions. This statement is not meant to diminish the importance of the parent groups; they should be provided with financial support to continue their needed educational activities.

In summary, an organized program for dealing with Sudden Infant Death Syndrome is mandatory in each and every community in the United States. None of the recommendations above require massive outlays of funds. Finding the cause and prevention of SIDS may be many years away and further augmentation of the research effort is imperative. However, a relatively modest investment in alleviating the discouraging psychological aspects of this all too human tragedy would produce remarkable changes for the better in a very short period of time.

CURRENT CLASSIFICATIONS OF PRIMARY COUNTIES IN EACH STANDARD METROPOLITAN STATISTICAL AREA (SMSA) WITH REFERENCE TO MANAGEMENT OF SIDS CASES*

Excellent Management

Sacramento, California
San Diego, California
Orleans, Louisiana
(New Orleans)
Baltimore, Maryland
Hennepin, Minnesota
(Minneapolis)
St. Louis, Missouri (County)
Multnomah, Oregon
(Portland)
Allegheny, Pennsylvania
(Pittsburgh)
King, Washington
(Seattle-Everett)

Good Management

Broome, New York
(Binghamton)
Erie, New York (Buffalo)
Nassau, New York
Cuyahoga, Ohio (Cleveland)
Philadelphia, Pennsylvania
Dallas, Texas
La Crosse, Wisconsin
Milwaukee, Wisconsin

Fair Management

Alameda, California
(Oakland)

San Francisco, California
Santa Clara, California
(San Jose)
San Joaquin, California
(Stockton)
Denver, Colorado
Hartford, Connecticut
Washington, D.C.
Dade, Florida (Miami)
Marion, Indiana
(Indianapolis)
Jefferson, Kentucky
(Louisville)
Yellowstone, Montana
(Billings)
Wayne, Michigan (Detroit)
Hillsborough, New Hampshire
(Manchester-Nashua)
Bergen, New Jersey
(Patterson-Clifton-Passaic)
Essex, New Jersey (Newark)
Brooklyn, New York
Ector, Texas (Odessa)
Harris, Texas (Houston)
Midland, Texas
Weber, Utah (Ogden)
Prince William, Virginia
Kenosha, Wisconsin

* Classifications are those of summer, 1972. Many improvements have subsequently occurred.

Generally Poor Management

Jefferson, Alabama
(Birmingham)
Montgomery, Alabama
Mobile, Alabama
Pulaski, Arkansas
(Little Rock)
Los Angeles, California
Orange, California
(Anaheim-Garden Grove)
San Bernadino, California
San Mateo, California
Alachua, Florida
(Gainesville)
Hillsborough, Florida
(Tampa-St. Petersburg)
Palm Beach, Florida
Fulton, Georgia (Atlanta)
Ada, Idaho (Boise)
Cook, Illinois (Chicago)
Winnebago, Illinois
(Rockford)
Vigo, Indiana (Terre Haute)
Wyandotte, Kansas
(Kansas City)
Bristol, Massachusetts
(New Bedford)

Suffolk, Massachusetts
(Boston)
Worcester, Massachusetts
(Fitchburg-Leominster)
Genessee, Michigan (Flint)
Ingham, Michigan (Lansing)
Kalamazoo, Michigan
Boone, Missouri (Columbia)
St. Louis, Missouri (city only)
New York, New York
Franklin, Ohio (Columbus)
Hamilton, Ohio (Cincinnati)
Jefferson, Ohio
(Steubenville-Wierton)
Comanche, Oklahoma
(Lawton)
Richland, South Carolina
(Columbia)
Davidson, Tennessee
(Nashville)
Cameron, Texas
(Brownsville-Harlingen-
San Benito)
Potter, Texas (Amarillo)
Utah, Utah (Provo)

SOME SMALLER COUNTIES MERIT HONORABLE MENTION

The smaller counties listed below deserve mention for the humane management of SIDS by county officials and health professionals. In each case, autopsies are encouraged by medical examiners and/or coroners and performed fairly routinely. SIDS or crib death is the common terminology on death certificates. Notification procedures are generally good; and in each county there is, at the very least, an informal channel of referral to other SIDS parents.

Middlesex County,
   Connecticut
Westchester County,
   New York
Niagara County, New York
Pinellas County, Florida

Marin County, California
Snohomish County,
   Washington
Clackamas County, Oregon
Du Page County, Illinois

THREE OUTSTANDING COMMUNITIES

The management of Sudden Infant Death Syndrome doesn't necessarily depend upon the qualifications or the credentials of those people within the legal and medical system who deal with the parents. Rather, it depends almost entirely on the compassion and the humanity of health professionals, medical examiners, coroners, and police. Along with several other communities in the United States, Baltimore, San Diego, and Orleans Parish (in Louisiana) have outstanding medical examiners/coroners and programs for dealing with this major health problem.

Dr. Russell S. Fisher, the State of Maryland's Chief Medical Examiner, is a distinguished forensic pathologist, who has had a long-time interest in SIDS research. Sudden infant death throughout the state of Maryland is managed on a statewide basis. Deputy medical examiners in each of the state's counties are appointed by Dr. Fisher and each deputy understands that all possible SIDS cases are to be reported to Dr. Fisher's office in Baltimore where autopsies are performed on all cases. Following the performance of the autopsy, Dr. Fisher's office informs the Baltimore-based Guild for Infant Survival, who in turn send a letter over Fisher's signature to new SIDS parents. The medical examiner's letter explains SIDS, stressing the unpredictability and unpreventability of the disease. The letter includes the names and phone number of a Guild member for the parent to contact for further counseling and assistance.

The county coroner of San Diego, California, Mr. Robert Creason, is a layman. Mr. Creason has had a long association with the San Diego-based chapter of the National Foundation for Sudden Infant Death. Like procedures followed in Maryland, all babies are autopsied and SIDS is used on the death certificates. Parents are promptly notified of the autopsy findings and sent an SIDS fact sheet and letter of condolence by Mr. Creason. In addition, Creason refers all SIDS parents to the San Diego parent group for further help.

Dr. Carl Rabin, an internist, is the Coroner of Orleans Parish (New Orleans), Louisiana. Louisiana law doesn't make autopsies mandatory; however, Dr. Rabin always has them performed on cases of sudden death of infants at New Orleans' Charity Hospital. Wherever applicable, the term "Sudden Infant Death Syndrome" has been ordered used as the official cause on the death certificates in the parish. As in Seattle, specially trained public health nurses are sent to the homes of SIDS families to counsel the parents. New Orleans and Seattle were the first two cities in the United States where the county health department became actively involved in dealing with SIDS parents. The New Orleans Chapter of NFSID is active in the community and along with Dr. Rabin's office and the parish health department, a coordinated effort to reach SIDS parents with the basic facts about the disease has been very successful.

There are other communities where the management of SIDS is outstanding. Seattle, Washington has served as a model community for many years. Minneapolis, Pittsburgh, Sacramento, Portland, and the county of St. Louis in Missouri, all have excellent medical examiners or coroners, who have teamed up with committed physicians and parents to create enlightened communities.

It seems clear that the tragic aftermath of sudden infant death can be somewhat relieved when the legal and medical professions are compassionate and responsive to the needs of the surviving family.

The state of Oregon probably has the best organized statewide system for the management of sudden infant death in the entire country. Due to the efforts of Chief Medical Investigator Dr. William Brady and his chief deputy, Dr. Larry Lewman, who are both forensic pathologists, Oregon has developed efficient and humane procedures. The state pays the salaries of the medical investigators in counties with populations in excess of 50,000. The pathologists are appointed by a State Board of Medical Examiners, which has statutory authority. The board is made up of persons such as the Professor of Pathology at the Medical School, the State Health Director and the President of the State Medical Association.

In addition to being responsible for the performance of autopsies in their home counties, the medical investigators provide consultation services to all other counties which require the services of a forensic pathologist. The Portland office reviews the death certificates from all other jurisdictions. A teletype system has been set up from the coroner's offices throughout the state to the Chief Medical Investigator's office in Portland.

Under Oregon law, each county in the state has a County Medical Examiner, who must be a physician. The county medical examiners are closely advised by Drs. Brady and Lewman in Portland. Autopsies are routinely performed on all cases of sudden infant death in the state and the diagnosis is teletyped to Portland immediately. Each medical examiner has copies of the NFSID brochure to send to parents as well as a letter from Dr. Lewman expressing condolences and offering the name of another SIDS parent in the community. At the same time, the state office sends a copy of the teletype to the president of the NFSID chapter in the state for further follow-up.

Suffolk County, Massachusetts which includes the greater Boston metropolitan area, has several world-famous medical centers within its environs. In 1972 Boston was an example of a poorly handled community in terms of sudden infant death. In 1970–71, about 32% of the potential SIDS cases were autopsied. The low autopsy rate was explained as due to the limitation of funds, facilities and personnel. In addition, medical examiners felt that the autopsy results had been "discouraging," though autopsies were performed if families or their private physicians insisted.

Acute pneumonitis, pulmonary congestion and interstitial pneumonitis are the most common terms, though occasionally sudden unexpected death at infancy is put in parentheses following the "official" designation. There was no standard notification procedure, though a provisional diagnosis is made within 24 hours of the gross autopsy. Parents ordinarily had to take the initiative to learn the results of that autopsy.

The Eastern Massachusetts chapter of the NFSID reaches relatively few families in Suffolk County; their main sphere of activity is in the Boston suburbs. A large number of poor SIDS families in the immediate Boston area got neither help nor counseling from the medical examiner's office or the NFSID.

PARENTS IN JAIL

The jailing of parents of a crib death victim as a result of their baby's death, while rare, does happen from time to time. Occasionally, overzealous law enforcement officials, always on the lookout for child abuse, charge and jail SIDS parents. The tragedy of SIDS is compounded many times over by such callous and barbaric treatment. Those unfortunate parents having to face this ordeal represent a small percentage of the approximately 10,000 families who lost babies last year. This tip of the iceberg, however, is indicative of the ignorance about SIDS in the United States. We would far rather "miss" a deliberate homicide than falsely suggest to a single SIDS mother that she might somehow have contributed to her baby's death. We've hopefully come a long way since 13th century Germany where, under penalty of law, parents were forbidden to allow a child under two years of age to sleep in the same bed with them, or 19th century Britain where a similar law was suggested. And yet in the 1970's, cases of incarcerated parents do crop up now and again. "Far too often an infant death in a 'nice' family is SIDS, but in other families, an identical kind of death is interpreted as suffocation, neglect or deliberate infanticide," Dr. Beckwith says. In each of the cases cited, the parents were young and poor and the charges against them were eventually dropped, but not after a prolonged period of mental anguish as the aura of suspicion surrounded them.

*   *   *   *

Roy and Evelyn Williams of New York City are young and black. In February 1971, Evelyn gave birth to the couple's second child, a son by caesarian section. Roy was home from the Army and taking care of the two children while Evelyn was undergoing out-patient psychiatric treatment for post-partum depression. On the morning of April 4, when the baby was two months old, Roy found him dead in his crib. The distraught parents spent about three hours cleaning their apartment before calling the police because they feared they'd be accused of some wrongdoing.

When the police were called, the baby's body was taken

to the hospital, the older child was left with a grandmother and the Williams' were taken to the police station. Roy and Evelyn were questioned separately for several hours. The policeman questioning Roy understood him to say that the baby hadn't been fed for three days—a statement Roy denied making.

An autopsy was performed by the deputy chief medical examiner. The diagnosis was listed as "congestion of the viscera" and the cause of death, "pending further study." In the autopsy report, there was no mention of malnutrition or dehydration. The medical examiner had inserted in the report the words "abandonment and neglect." On the basis of the police and medical examiner's reports, the parents were brought before a grand jury and indicted on charges of "criminal neglect." The family is poor and was not able to raise the $1,000 bond, so on June 4, 1971, they went to jail. Roy spent five months and his wife six months in New York City jails, until the bail was finally raised by relatives.

Their case came to trial in May 1972. The medical examiner testified that he'd written "abandonment and neglect" on his report based solely on his conversation with the police and *not* as a result of his post-mortem findings. Further, he stated in court that his findings were "consistent with crib death."

At the conclusion of the prosecution's case, the judge dismissed the charges. Evelyn and Roy Williams' ordeal with the law was over, they were free. More than 19 months after their baby son's death, they were free to live with the horror of having spent half a year inside jails mourning for an infant who was a victim of SIDS.

* * * *

John Jerry and Billy Mae Price of Fort Mill, South Carolina are white, poor and illiterate. In July 1972, the couple lost their second child to SIDS. Autopsy findings on their six-month-old son indicated that he was a victim of SIDS. Nevertheless, John Jerry was thrown into jail before the post-mortem findings were available on a charge of "assault and battery with intent to kill." Billy Mae, mercifully, was released from jail when it was learned she was not at home the night the baby died. John pleaded with the authorities at the jail to allow him to attend his baby's funeral, in chains, if necessary. He was refused. At first the family was told they would have to raise $150.00 bail but when they arrived at the jail with the money, they were told the bond was in fact $1,500, a sum way out of their reach.

Several days later, the medical examiner's office informed the county police that there was no indication whatever that the baby had been abused in any way. It was the medical examiner's opinion that the baby had died of SIDS. John Jerry was still not released from jail because the police insisted they had to have a release order in writing before they could let him go. At the time, the young parents had very little idea of what had happened to them, "I don't think they treated us right at all," John said, "it was bad enough to lose the baby . . . and then to be locked up . . ." Billie Mae was sure of one thing, though, she wouldn't have any more children—"No, not if I can help it. I had two and couldn't raise those two, so there ain't no use in having them."

* * * *

Patricia and John Smiley of Elsinore, California are also young and poor. John is 21 and his wife is 20. In the early morning hours of April 11, 1973, they put their month-old daughter to sleep in an extended dresser drawer—they couldn't afford a crib. Later in the day, they found their baby lifeless. John, who is a hospital orderly, called the Riverside county sheriff's office for help. Because of the run-down condition of the Smiley's apartment, the police suspected child neglect. John and Patricia were taken to jail and charged with "involuntary manslaughter" even before an autopsy was performed. The parents remained in jail for two days until the $2000 bail was posted by John's mother. At no time, during the period when they were charged and arraigned on April 17, did they have a lawyer. The National Foundation for Sudden Infant Death, upon hearing of the Smiley's plight, retained an attorney in Riverside and members of the Board of Trustees personally contributed the money to defray the costs of the young couple's defense.

At the preliminary hearing, the prosecution alleged that the baby had been neglected, but there was no evidence whatsoever to substantiate the charge. The Smileys were guilty of being poor and young; too poor to afford a crib for the baby. The autopsy findings were reviewed by an independent pathologist and the results were found to be consistent with sudden infant death. As a result of those findings, the official charges were dropped and like the others, John and Patricia Smiley were free to live with their memories of time spent behind bars, official accusations, and a legal hearing while grieving over the death of their baby daughter.

X

EPILOGUE

Our epilogue was written by Colman McCarthy of *The Washington Post*. Mr. McCarthy wrote the following editorial on September 21, 1973 following a hearing on federal legislation (S. 1745) before the Senate Subcommittees on (1) Children and Youth and (2) Health. He says, from an "outsider's" viewpoint, all there is to say on the state of the problem. We can only hope that an editorial such as this will not have to be written in 1983. We have made our commitment to future families; we are waiting for others to follow.

"The Tragedy of Crib Death"
Colman McCarthy

Earlier this year in a small California town near San Diego, John and Patricia Smiley went into the bedroom of their four week old infant. The child, healthy the day before, lay dead. The couple, frantic with sudden shock, immediately called the local sheriff's office to ask for an ambulance. As Smiley remembers it, the voice at the other end replied that if the child was dead, why was an ambulance needed.

So began the post-death ordeal of the Smileys. The young and poor couple was charged on suspicion of involuntary manslaughter and jailed for three days. The charges were eventually dropped but not before the couple had been harrassed to the point that they left town. The Smileys were in Washington yesterday, testifying before a joint session of

127

the Senate subcommittee on children and youth and the subcommittee on health. "There are just so many bad memories to the whole situation and I would like to forget," Smiley told the senators, "but I know that I will never be able to forget . . . I hope that it never happens to anyone else like it happened to us. The death of a child is bad enough. It's the harrassment and lack of knowledge, lack of understanding and lack of compassion that hurts more than anything else."

The tragedy of the Smileys would pass unnoticed—another hard luck case in a world full of them—except that it is part of a national pattern. Their child died from Sudden Infant Death Syndrome, a disease that kills an estimated 10,000 infants a year, at a ratio of one in 350. SIDS (crib death) is neither predictable nor preventable. Perhaps because of this, interest in its research has been limited, from medical schools to the federal government; current federal primary money for SIDS research grants is $262,000, less than the cost of remodeling the President's jet; primary research contracts are $340,000. What is especially strange about the disease is not its mystery but that little is done for the surviving parents, even though much is known about their anguish. Couples are not usually jailed as the Smileys were, but nearly all are imprisoned within some kind of emotional torment from which release is painful and perhaps impossible.

Many who are concerned about SIDS learned long ago not to look to the federal government for leadership, much less to local health officials. Instead, several private groups are at work. Among them are the Guild for Infant Survival (Baltimore) and the National Foundation for Sudden Infant Death (New York). In testimony yesterday, Dr. Abraham Bergman, a Seattle pediatrician and the foundation's presi-

dent, said that the parents' post-death anguish "is all so unnecessary. By the expenditure of a small amount of funds
(such as proposed in legislation now before the Senate),
and just the semblance of some action on the part of HEW,
the human aspects of SIDS which causes an enormous toll
of mental illness could be solved within two years."

In other years, Bergman has come to Washington with
mostly general statements on the degree of neglect. The response was small. This time, he is presenting specific details
from 158 American communities on what action coroners,
medical examiners, health officials and parents take when
infants die suddenly and unexpectedly. The report, with a
few bright parts, is generally bleak. A coroner in Alabama
called a SIDS death suffocation because "blacks do not know
how to care for their children properly." An Idaho coroner
called it "partial neglect and pneumonia." Only half of some
400 parents were told their children died of SIDS. Only 27
per cent of the communities had pathologists to certify the
cause of death; in 43 per cent of the communities it was not
even a physician who performed this service, but often an
undertaker, ambulance driver or sheriff. More than a third
of the families had to wait between a week and many months
before the autopsy results were provided; 9 per cent were
never told by anyone why their infants died.

Not surprisingly, Bergman's study found racial and class
discrimination in the management of SIDS. "Half as many
blacks as whites were given SIDS as an explanation for
death; four times as many blacks were told that their baby
suffocated; and three times more blacks than whites were
never told why their baby died. Some 75 per cent of upper
class families had heard of SIDS before their baby died, and
92 per cent received information afterwards. Only 48 per
cent of lower-class families had heard of SIDS before their

baby died and only 40 per cent received information about SIDS after their baby died. The people who needed the help most were least apt to receive it."

The loss of an infant causes an anguish that only the surviving parents can feel. Even when a parent is familiar with the disease, the trauma can be intense. A Seattle pediatrician working in the hospital with the world's largest SIDS research project said that her knowledge that SIDS is neither predictable nor preventable ". . . . did not protect me from painful guilt feelings and depression. I was a human being and a mother who needed help at a critical time." She was visiting in Los Angeles when her infant son died and the help was not provided. More than two months passed before she even knew that an autopsy had been performed. "I keep thinking," the woman has written, "if a physician's family, which has some understanding of SIDS, is treated in this way in Los Angeles, what happens to other families who don't have similiar resources? Why can't parents who lose treasured infants be treated with dignity and compassion?"

It is a fair question. One possible answer is the lack of leadership among public health officials. Why should a local sheriff's office be expected to show sensitivity if no example is given by the supposedly alert doctors in many state and federal agencies? At the last Senate hearings on SIDS, an HEW doctor in charge of SIDS research issued the inevitable promise to take action, but he's gone from the agency now. His successor has renewed the promise. "I don't know what happens to people when they come back here to the banks of the Potomac," Bergman said. "Maybe it's the heat or maybe it's the smog. Government officials here in Washington are always busy, busy with *big problems*. HEW always seems to have some reorganization cooking. *Global* health strategy is being devised, or else 'we're new in our job, just give us time.' Senator Magnuson says that, what with all the job changes, the busiest people in this town are the sign painters down at HEW."

If we were told this morning that in the next year a dreadful plague would kill 10,000 of America's children, it is likely the nation's medical community would command the front pages of newspapers to announce plans to meet the threat. The sign painters at HEW would be idle because no official would dare leave his post in this emergency. Every local community, including Alabama coroners, would be on the alert. Such a plague is not coming, of course, at least not the Black Death kind of threat. But a year from now, another 10,000 infants will have been found dead in their cribs. Afterward, their parents will die repeated emotional deaths in private anguish. The research to prevent SIDS may be far off, but ways to prevent the abuse of surviving parents is well known. Perhaps the largest mystery involving SIDS is that we are not acting on facts already available.

APPENDIX

Question	Number Responding	% Yes	% No
Was an autopsy performed?	414	74	24
Was permission requested?	372	64	36
Was verbal explanation of diagnosis same as that appearing on death certificate?	310	66	33
Was cause of death adequately explained?	389	50	50
Was a coroner's inquest held?	395	3	97
Was a private physician involved?	337	68	32
Did anyone outside family offer assistance after baby's death?	405	78	22
Did you know anything about SIDS before the death?	415	58	42
Have you had access to printed material about SIDS?	415	74	26

PARENT INTERVIEWS
DID ANY PERSON OR PERSONS MAKE THE SITUATION WORSE?

	Number Responding	No Percent	YES *Percent of those who "made it worse"
No one made it worse	202	49	51
"Friends"	58	14	28
Physicians or nurses	43	11	21
Relatives	41	10	20
Policemen	15	4	7
Newspaper story	8	2	4
Firemen	2	.3	1
Other persons	40	9.7	19
Total Responses	409		

* Of the 51% who made things worse, numerical total (N), 207.

PARENT INTERVIEWS

WHAT DO YOU NOW THINK WAS THE CAUSE OF YOUR CHILD'S DEATH?

	Number Responding	Percent
SIDS or crib death	262	64*
Don't know	56	13.5
Pneumonia	21	5.1
Crib death with "contributing factors"	16	4*
Suffocation	14	3.5
Some infection	2	.7
Other	38	9.2
Total Responses	409	

* Combined percentages, 68%.

PARENT INTERVIEWS

HAD YOU EVER HEARD OF SIDS PRIOR TO YOUR BABY'S DEATH?

	Percent
Yes	58
No	42
Those who possessed information obtained it from: (231 responses)	
Magazine article	19
Newspaper story	18
"Word of mouth"	15
Television	7
Combination of above	17
Other	24

PARENT INTERVIEWS

WHAT PRINTED MATERIAL HELPED YOU AT THE TIME OF YOUR BABY'S DEATH?

	Number Responding	Percent
NFSID brochure	77	19
Newspaper or magazine story	67	16
Both of above	111	27
Other	49	12
I had no printed material	106	26
Total Responses	410	

PARENT INTERVIEWS
SOCIAL CLASS DISTRIBUTION BY OCCUPATION OF
345 FAMILIES RESPONDING

		Number Responding
Class I	Professional and managerial	143
Class II	Skilled workers and clerical	127
Class III	Unskilled laborers and unemployed	75

PARENT INTERVIEWS
RELATIONSHIP OF SOCIAL CLASS TO INFORMATION
RECEIVED ABOUT CAUSE OF BABY'S DEATH

	Class			
	I	II	III	Overall
Autopsy rate	75%	77%	70%	74%
Private physician involved	77	74	49	73
Families *initiating* contact to receive autopsy results	34	29	41	32
Cause of death adequately explained	56	50	34	50
Previous knowledge of SIDS	75	57	48	63
Received printed information	92	78	40	79

PARENT INTERVIEWS
PERCENTAGES OF FAMILIES HAVING ACCESS TO PRINTED MATERIAL
ON SIDS BEFORE AND AFTER CHILD'S DEATH BY SOCIAL CLASS

	Class			
	I	II	III	Overall
Knowledge of SIDS before death	75%	57%	48%	63%
Number of responses	106	155	46	307
Received printed material about SIDS after death	92%	78%	40%	79%
Number of responses	141	154	48	343

PARENT INTERVIEWS
RELATIONSHIP OF SOCIAL CLASS TO THE PERSON
FOUND MOST HELPFUL AFTER CHILD'S DEATH

| | Class | | | |
	I	II	III	Overall
Member of own family	37%	33%	66%	42%
Family physician	19	20	7	17
Clergyman	9	19	3	8
Parent group	10	8	—	6
Coroner/medical examiner	2	8	3	4
Other person	23	12	21	23
Number responding	139	154	47	340

PARENT INTERVIEWS
PERCENTAGE OF FAMILIES IN EACH SOCIAL CLASS
RECEIVING PARTICULAR EXPLANATION FOR CHILD'S DEATH

| | Class | | | |
	I	II	III	Overall
SIDS or crib death	63%	57%	45%	52%
Pneumonia	9	15	14	14
Suffocation or strangulation	2	7	9	4
Other	20	14	15	16
No explanation	6	7	17	14
Number responding	142	155	48	345

PARENT INTERVIEWS
PERCENTAGE OF FAMILIES IN EACH SOCIAL CLASS
CONCEPT OF CHILD'S DEATH AT TIME OF INTERVIEW

| | Class | | | |
	I	II	III	Overall
SIDS or crib death	84%	67%	57%	73%
Suffocation or strangulation	—	4	9	3
Other	10	14	17	12
Don't know	6	15	17	12
Number responding	139	154	46	339

PARENT INTERVIEWS
RACIAL DISTRIBUTION

	Number Responding	Percent
Caucasian	329	79
Black	66	16
Mexican-American	15	4
American Indian	1	—
Other/unknown	7	1
Total Responding	418	

PARENT INTERVIEWS
RACIAL DIFFERENCES IN MANAGEMENT OF SIDS

	Number Responding	Response Rate (%) Caucasian	Black
Private physician involved	337	76	35
Policeman involved	413	35	48
Fireman involved	413	24	6

PARENT INTERVIEWS
RACIAL DIFFERENCES IN MANAGEMENT OF SIDS

	Number Responding	Response Rate (%) Caucasian	Black
Permission requested to perform autopsy	370	68	45
Adequate information given on cause of death	415	57	27
No information provided on cause of death	411	5	23
Assistance provided	403	85	53

Qualifications of 138 Public Officials Certifying
Cause of Death

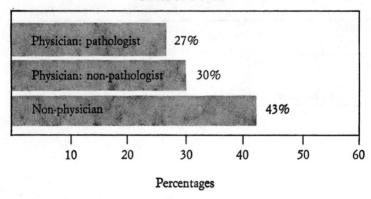

Percentages

What is the Usual Length of Time After Performance of an
Autopsy When a Diagnosis is Entered on the
Death Certificate?
Responses of 137 Coroners or Medical Examiners

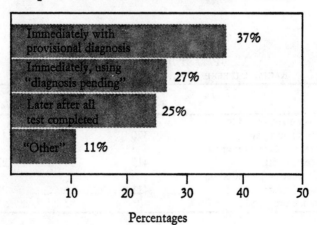

Percentages

Who Was The First "Official" Person With Whom You Had Contact After Discovering Infant?

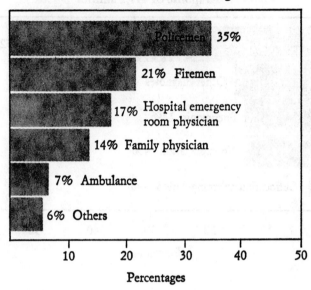

Policemen 35%

21% Firemen

17% Hospital emergency room physician

14% Family physician

7% Ambulance

6% Others

Percentages

Where Was Body Taken Following Discovery In Home? Responses of 417 Families

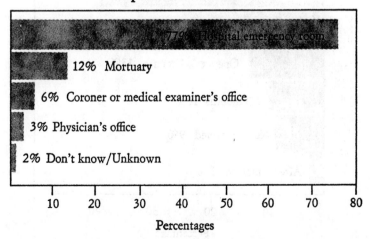

77% Hospital emergency room

12% Mortuary

6% Coroner or medical examiner's office

3% Physician's office

2% Don't know/Unknown

Percentages

What Explanation Were You Given About The Cause of Death? Response of 417 Families

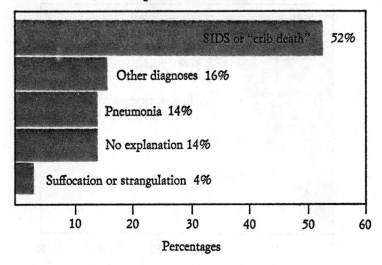

SIDS or "crib death" 52%

Other diagnoses 16%

Pneumonia 14%

No explanation 14%

Suffocation or strangulation 4%

10   20   30   40   50   60

Percentages

How Long After The Autopsy Did You Learn the Results? Responses of 413 Families

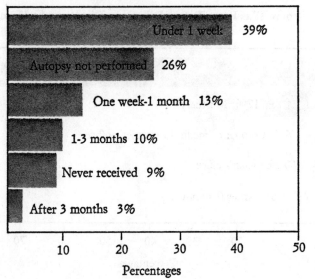

Under 1 week 39%

Autopsy not performed 26%

One week-1 month 13%

1-3 months 10%

Never received 9%

After 3 months 3%

10   20   30   40   50

Percentages

Who Was *Most* Helpful To You After Baby's Death?
Responses of 409 Families

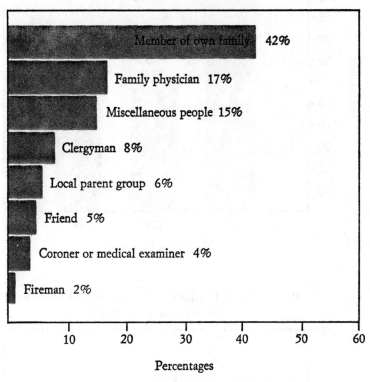

Member of own family   42%

Family physician   17%

Miscellaneous people   15%

Clergyman   8%

Local parent group   6%

Friend   5%

Coroner or medical examiner   4%

Fireman   2%

10   20   30   40   50   60

Percentages

Percentage of Families Having Knowledge of SIDS Before Death

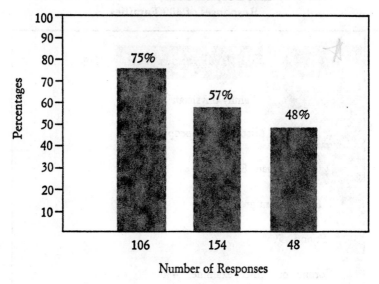

Number of Responses

Percentage of Families Who Received Information About SIDS After Death

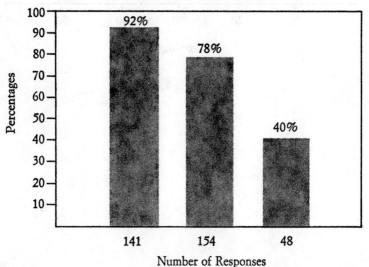

Number of Responses

Length of Time to Receive Autopsy Results
Relationship of Race

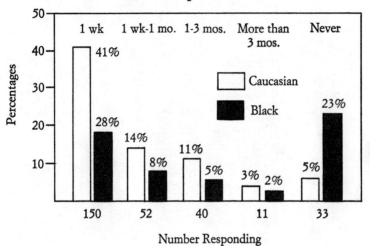

Number Responding

Relationship of Race to Explanation of Cause of Death

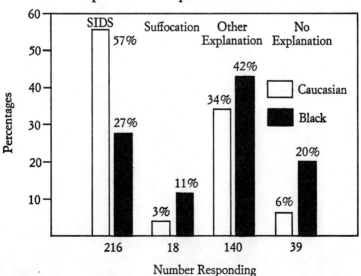

Number Responding

Bibliography

1. Adelson, L. and Kinney, E. R.: "Sudden and Unexpected Death in Infancy and Childhood," *Pediatrics*, 17:663, 1956.

2. Beckwith, J. B. and Bergman, A. B.: "The Sudden Death Syndrome of Infancy," *Hospital Practice*, 2:44, 1967.

3. Beckwith, J. B.: "The Sudden Infant Death Syndrome, *Current Problems in Pediatrics*," Vol. III, No. 8, June 1973 (Yearbook Medical Publishers, Inc., Chicago, Illinois).

4. Bergman, A. B., Miller, J. D. and Beckwith, J. B.: "Sudden Death Syndrome: The Physician's Role, *Clinical Pediatrics*," 5:711, 1966.

5. Bergman, A. B., Pomeroy, M. A. and Beckwith, J. B.: "The Psychiatric Toll of SIDS," *General Practice*, 40:99-105, 1969.

6. Bergman, A. B., Beckwith, J. B. and Ray, C. G. (eds.) *Proceedings of the Second International Conference on Causes of Sudden Death in Infants* (Seattle: University of Washington Press, 1970).

7. Bergman, A. B., Ray, C. G., Pomeroy, M. A., Wahl, P. W. and Beckwith, J. B.: "Studies of the Sudden Infant Death Syndrome in King County, Washington; III Epidemiology, *Pediatrics*, 49:860, 1972.

8. Bergman, A. B.: "I Practice Political Medicine," *Puget Soundings*, May 1973.

9. Bergman, A. B.: *A Study in the Management of SIDS—Summer 1972* (NFSID, New York, 1973).

10. Cadden, V.: "Why Babies Die," *Redbook*, November 1963.

11. Gold, E., Adelson, L. and Goldek, G.: "The Role of Antibody to Cow's Milk Proteins with the Sudden Death Syndrome, *Pediatrics*, 33:541, 1964.

12. LeBlanc, R. D.: "Somebody Help My Baby!", *Good Housekeeping*, July 1973.

13. Peterson, D. R.: "Sudden Unexpected Death in Infants: Incidence in Two Climatically Dissimilar Metropolitan Communities, *American Journal of Epidemiology*, 95:95, 1972.

14. Pomeroy, M. A.: "Sudden Death Syndrome," *American Journal of Nursing*, 69:1886-1891, September 1969.

15. Ray, C. G. *et al*: "Studies of the Sudden Infant Death Syndrome in King County, Washington: I. The role of viruses, *JAMA* 211:619, 1970.

16. *Rights of Children, 1972, "Hearing Before the Subcommittee on Children and Youth of the Committee on Labor and Public Welfare, U.S. Senate,"* 92nd Congress, Jan. 25, 1972, U.S. Gov't Printing Office, Washington, D.C.

17. Szybist, C.: *The Subsequent Child* (NFSID, New York, 1973).

18. Templeman, C.: "258 Cases of Suffocation in Infants," *Edinburgh Medical Journal*, 38:322, 1893.

19. Valdes-Dapena, M.: "Sudden and Unexpected Death in Infants: The Scope of our Ignorance," *Pediatric Clinics of North America*, August 1963.

20. Valdes-Dapena, M., Birle, L. J., McGovern, J. A. McGillen, J. F. and Colwell, F. H.: "Sudden Unexpected Death in Infancy: A Statistical Analysis of Certain Socio-economic Factors," *Journal of Pediatrics*, Vol. 73, No. 3, 387-394, September 1968.

21. Wedgwood, R. J. and Benditt, E. P. (eds.) *Proceedings of the Conference on Causes of Sudden Death in Infants* (PHS Pub. No. 1412, U.S. Gov't Printing Office, Washington, D.C., 1963).

22. Wooley, P. V.: "Mechanical Suffocation during Infancy: A Comment on its Relation to the Total Problem of Sudden Death," *Journal of Pediatrics*, 26:572, 1945.

23. Froggatt, P., Lynas, M. A. and Marshall, T. K.: "Sudden Unexpected Death in Infants ("cot death"): Report of a Collaborative Study in Northern Ireland," *Ulster M. J.*, 40:116, 1971.

24. Naeye, R. L.: "Pulmonary Arterial Abnormalities in the Sudden

Infant Death Syndrome, *New England Journal of Medicine*, 289:1167-1170, 1973.

25. Steinschneider, A.: "Prolonged Apnea and the Sudden Infant Death Syndrome; Clinical and Laboratory Observations," *Pediatrics*, 50:646-654, 1972.

INDEX

FIRST AID
IN
MENTAL HEALTH

By the same author
Phobias and Obsessions

FIRST AID
IN
MENTAL HEALTH

JOY MELVILLE

London
GEORGE ALLEN & UNWIN
Boston   Sydney

First published in 1980

GEORGE ALLEN & UNWIN LTD
40 Museum Street, London WC1A 1LU

British Library Cataloguing in Publication Data

Melville, Joy
   First aid in mental health.
   1. Psychiatry
   I. Title
   616.8'91   RC480   80-40856

   ISBN 0-04-362033-7
   ISBN 0-04-362034-5 Pbk

Set in 11 on 12 point Fournier by Bedford Typesetters Ltd
and printed in Great Britain
by Lowe & Brydone Ltd, Thetford, Norfolk

CONTENTS

AUTHOR'S ACKNOWLEDGEMENTS

A great many people, and organisations, have been helpful in the preparation of this book. I would particularly like to thank the Director and staff of MIND (the National Association for Mental Health), and especially Ron Lacey, for their advice and criticism.

INTRODUCTION

People discuss physical illness. They give advice, pass on suggestions, offer help. If they have not been affected by the particular illness, it is probable that someone they know has. There is usually concerned interest and open comment.

With mental disturbance it is different. It is less easily admitted – whether it concerns oneself or relatives – and is often greeted with embarrassment and unease. As one ex-psychiatric patient said: 'You don't make the mistake twice of telling people you've had electric shock treatment. Not after you see the way they look at you.'

The result of this reticence is that, when any form of mental disturbance occurs, people are both alarmed and ignorant. They do not know what sort of treatment is needed, or where to get it. A broken bone can only be mended in one way; a broken mind is different. It responds to different treatment. Many people do not know if treatment is even necessary: perhaps other people feel, or act this way? The doctor is thought of as someone who cures physical, not mental, illness.

The kind of problems which people faced with the onset of mental disturbance in themselves or others feel they need advice about can be seen from the letters and calls received by MIND (the National Association for Mental Health). In one randomly selected fortnight, for instance, some of the problems presented were:

A request by a woman wanting to know of any group for depressed people, like herself; a man needing help to deal with his tenant, who was behaving bizarrely; a woman with marital and individual problems, wanting somewhere to go to talk these over; a man with constant feelings of fear, wanting relief from these; a girl wanting to see a psychiatrist (uninvolved people may think this a simple problem, but I have frequently found that those concerned did not know where to go); a woman wanting treatment other than tranquillisers; a father wanting to know what to do with his deeply depressed and isolated son; a woman with a fear of getting cancer; a man worried about his mother and her developing dementia; an upset and confused young man wanting help; a sister worried about the side-effects of her brother's schizophrenia; a man wanting advice about his fears of going outside the house; help asked by a man who was living with his parents who were paranoid and would not visit the doctor (a cause of depression in younger people is having to look after elderly relatives and feeling trapped); a man wanting help to stop his panic attacks.

There was, in addition, one request for information on hypno-therapy, and one on group therapy. A man was concerned about his wife who had had a history of depression but was now behaving oddly; a woman, depressed after having her breast removed, wanted some kind of counselling help; a woman who had had private psycho-therapy for six months was now distressed and confused and unable to afford to continue her treatment; a woman was worried about her mother's nerve trouble. One ex-patient wanted to make a complaint about the hospital; another wanted long-stay accommodation of some kind. Quite a few social workers wanted help and advice about accommodation for patients leaving hospital. One girl wanted to know of a nearby day centre. A man was worried about his brother-in-law, a schizophrenic who was not receiving benefit money because his parents were too proud to claim (showing how people dislike having to admit to mental illness within their family circle). Another man asked if it was a mistake to tell people in general that he had been diagnosed schizophrenic; a woman wanted help to overcome her fear of being alone in the house; another woman was concerned about her brother who was suffering monthly periods of depression, lasting for a week; a man was worried about the job reference his psychiatrist might give him (sometimes a firm, on being told an applicant has had hospital treatment, contacts his medical practitioner, to check his condition).

These few selected examples give an idea of the range of problems arising from mental disturbance that many people find of concern and difficult to solve. Of the 600 or 700 people I have seen, or whose letters I have read, and who were upset, frightened or bewildered by mental disorder in themselves or their relations, two things stood out: the need for practical information on where to go for help, and reassurance that they were not alone in their problem. I have written this book in the hope that it will give assistance in precisely these areas of concern.

I

Warning Signs

The onset of mental disturbance can be so gradual that one may be unaware that anything is going wrong. It is, nevertheless, important to be able to recognise warning signs – the earlier treatment is started, the less likelihood there will be of admission to hospital. There is also the possibility that the symptoms mask a physical illness.

Early signals of mental ill-health will vary according to the particular illness and are illustrated in more detail in the specific chapters later in this book. But there are general changes in behaviour that act as a serious signal that something is wrong and help is needed. The case which follows illustrates how one girl's mental ill-health developed.

The girl concerned, in her early twenties, advertised for a flatmate. She told the girl who answered the advertisement that she wanted company, and had been seeing a psychiatrist for depression – a depression, she explained, which rendered her unable to tell the difference between a cold, snowy day and a warm, sunny one. Everything she saw seemed to be in black and white, with no colour.

For the first year or so that she was living there, the flatmate did not notice any change in the girl – though she went out as much as possible because she did find the girl rather depressing company. However, the girl seemed to improve after her psychiatrist decided to take her off all drugs. After two or three months, though, a gradual change took place in the girl's behaviour.

'It started with her obsessive tidyness,' said the flatmate. 'If I ate a biscuit, she would follow me round and tidy up the crumbs. Then she would move a biscuit from one plate to another and wash up the first plate. She would ask people to tea at weekends and buy masses of food, but stayed out in the kitchen herself, clattering away, washing the floor, and bringing in ever more food. If you said, "Come and sit down and have a cup of tea," she would get furious and say, "This is my flat, I'll do what I want, don't you boss me around." Although I was out quite late in the evenings, she'd still be up when I came in at midnight. She'd stay up till 4 a.m. ironing, or so she'd tell me the next morning. She would take an hour to iron a blouse, and would be in every evening, ironing, washing, sewing.'

The first really strange happening, in the flatmate's eyes, was when the girl announced that there was a poltergeist in the flat and that it had flung the clock over to the other side of the room. She wrote 'Hate, hate, hate' on her memory slate, and said that this, too, had been written by the poltergeist. Then she started writing on the walls and on the back of doors – one door was filled with the initials of the flatmate. She talked of 'them' and said that there was a conspiracy against her; by keeping the radio on very loud, she tried to drown out the voices menacing her. At one point she attached a rope from her bedroom door to the front door, writing on it 'keep out burglars', then tied some apple and cheese to the front door for, in her eyes, further protection.

The flatmate asked if she was telling the psychiatrist about her feelings of a conspiracy and the messages and, despite the reassurance from the girl that she had, suspected this was not the case. The flatmate did not like to interfere, although she was aware that it was only since the girl had been taken off her drugs to counteract depression some months previously that her behaviour had become increasingly bizarre.

'I would try to phone her during the day to make sure she was all right,' said the flatmate, 'but she would take the phone off the hook because she would sleep during the day and then wake up at night and want to talk at 3 a.m. She would talk very loudly, and play the gramophone loudly. I'd hear it even through my closed bedroom door. The neighbours were amazingly tolerant of the blare once they realised she was ill. I'd never know what to expect when I came home: whether she would be sprawled out asleep on a chair, or out, or "high". She wouldn't eat unless I prepared it for her and then she would gulp down an enormous plate in seconds. It couldn't have done her any good and she remained thin.

'She went out one day and bought nearly £300 worth of cosmetics; and another day she borrowed £5 to go to the supermarket, and came back with three or four bags and a supermarket wheeler absolutely full of large packets of soap powder and bread. She must have used her credit card. The food in the fridge began to go bad, but, when I tried to take out some fermenting yogurts that were absolutely brimming over, she said she might want them. The spin drier was full of mouldy clothes, and so was the washing machine. Then she bought a rabbit, locked her own bedroom door, and slept in a tiny room along with the rabbit. The smell became awful, right through the flat. Her room was full of muesli, rabbit leavings, lettuce, piles of clothes, old bread, train tickets – once I saw five train tickets all to the same place in Surrey, all dated the same day. She must have gone back and forward all day long.'

At this stage, the flatmate felt that she could cope no longer. She went to the girl's own doctor to explain the situation. Although he could not, ethically, discuss a patient, both he and the area psychiatrist considered that the girl should be compulsorily admitted to psychiatric hospital. The girl had no relations, and it required a social worker to agree to the compulsory admittance (*see Chapter 9 on patient's rights*). The flatmate was told that the social worker was coming to see her and, when she did, behaved very calmly. Although the social worker agreed the girl was very thin, and saw the writing on the walls, she put the girl down as hyperactive and would not sign the compulsory order. When she left, said the flatmate, the girl 'burst into hysterical laughter and said, "That wasn't a social worker." '

After that, nothing happened. The flatmate felt she could not leave as there was no one to look after the girl, but became progressively exhausted and depressed herself. Her work was disrupted by phone calls from the girl, and so was her sleep at night. But as the girl would not accept that she was mentally ill, or go into hospital voluntarily, or see the doctor, there was no way to give her treatment. Only after she left the flat and started staying in hotels, running up, over some two months, large bills which she could not pay, was a compulsory order signed.

GENERAL SIGNS

Many of the signs of growing mental ill-health are much less noticeable
than the case above. A member of the family, for instance, who is
normally active at weekends, may start lying in bed all morning – and
this will then begin to extend to weekdays. Or he may change from
spending a reasonable time in the bath to lying in it for two or three
hours. Sometimes a person who was formerly neat and tidy may
cease bothering to put things away and start to neglect her appearance.
Or someone will become more and more withdrawn, staying for long
periods in his room and rarely speaking to others in the family. One
woman said, 'For many weeks now, I have done nothing but sit alone in
my room. I have no inclination to find work or take part in any social
activities. I do not seem to have an interest in anything and have more
or less lost touch with my family and friends. I have almost lost the
will to go on living and have no sense of purpose whatsoever.'

Patterns of waking and sleeping can also change. One mother said,
'My son would not tell me what was wrong. But he just stayed in bed
all day and stayed up at night.' And a teenager, talking of her father,
said, 'He wakes at about 4 a.m., and walks about the house, then falls
asleep in the chair as soon as he returns from work.'

Occasionally, a person's character seems to go into reverse: quiet
people may become aggressive; the extroverts may become withdrawn. It is puzzling and worrying for relatives. 'My middle-aged son
becomes very manic and overactive at times,' said one woman. 'But this
wild behaviour must be a cry for help; he is by nature the opposite of
violent or aggressive. He is demoralised by this condition and I fear
will get more and more subject to these episodes, if only as a means
of escaping from what he cannot cope with in ordinary life.'

A girl, in talking of her brother, said: 'There has been a great change
in his personality. He gets into a terrible temper about the slightest
little thing I or anyone does that annoys him. All his friends have
fallen away. He was always houseproud, but now the flat is neglected
and he seems unaware of how dirty it is. I tried to tell him he was ill,
but he flew into a terrible temper and said he was all right.'

'My teenage daughter, who was always shy and withdrawn, now

has outbursts of temper,' another woman said. 'She stays up in the chair all night and goes to bed at 7 a.m. She's full of obsessions, always looking at her clothes and hands, vacuuming the bedroom for hours, and will not have the door open.'

Constant tears are an obvious sign that a person is not coping. 'I can be reading a book and, for no reason at all, I just burst out crying,' said one woman. Another, who mentioned that she too cried a lot and often thought that she was going mad because of her inexplicable feelings of fear, said that her friends and relatives were losing patience with her 'because I'm either crying or just can't make conversation, or sit without talking'.

One girl, whose boss sent her home on a number of occasions because she kept bursting into tears, could not understand what was the matter with herself. 'Nobody in our family had ever had a breakdown: I simply did not know it existed. I was living in a large house in Harrow with five other girls, one of whom I disliked intensely, and was very unhappy. None of them seemed to realise there was anything untoward in my behaviour. Yet, from what I remember, it was weird. For instance, I believed that my mother, who lived in the country, was up in London. My flatmates would get me to ring her, to prove that she was still in the country; but as soon as I rang off I would believe she was in London again. I also had a mania for writing everything down. It got to the point, where, if I told something to a flatmate, I would not believe she was listening, so I would write it all down and ask her to read it. I also began to think there were burglars in the house. I went shopping one morning, but had to come back because I thought all the shop assistants were against me.

'My mother was worried sick because she kept getting these peculiar, hysterical phone calls. But none of my flatmates said anything. I suppose ignorance was the answer. They had never come across it before and did not know how to deal with it.'

Shortly after this, the girl caught an infection, which brought matters to a climax. She went home, was lucid in the mornings, but became worse as the day wore on. She did not know the people around her, and imagined they were taping her conversations and following her around. She finally became violent and was admitted to hospital. She was told that had she been treated at the onset she would not have had such a severe breakdown.

The tension and stress that had triggered off this girl's condition were also present in another case, that of a schoolteacher. He was, at the time, a housemaster and had been given additional responsibility at school. He was also spending a great deal of time learning the organ. His wife was pregnant and, lacking enough money to decorate the house, they were doing so themselves. He became hyperactive, corresponding with eminent musicians, and becoming overexcited when dealing with colleagues, whom he was having difficulty in handling. Neither he nor his wife was aware of these warning signs. He began to get increasingly worked up; he saw sinister implications in the various political events of the day, and in the comings and goings of his colleagues. He began to have grave doubts about the merits of teaching at public school. When he happened to go on a train journey and came across a colleague on the same train, he thought it was all part of a conspiracy against him. Finally, at a dinner party he and his wife gave one evening, he became very disturbed and excited and, to the distress of his wife, broke it up. She suggested he should see a doctor, which he refused to accept. Only when a colleague suggested this did he do so. The doctor prescribed tranquillisers, but this did little good. The teacher remained disturbed all that day, and finally made an improper phone call to a girl he knew. He revisited the school, as he felt he needed further help from his colleagues, and the deputy headmaster persuaded him to become a voluntary patient in a psychiatric hospital.

In another case, a man was aware of the warning signs of mental disturbance. 'I knew two people who had breakdowns,' he said, 'and from knowing them I could see the signs in myself. They made me aware of oddities in myself, and made me think about things that I regarded as normal.' He realised, for instance, that he was avoiding certain situations. One example was dropping out of day classes, which his boss had given him permission to attend. His marriage had broken up, but his wife then had a bad motor accident. The strain of going to see her daily began to tell. He could not bear anyone to come near him. He would come in from work on Friday night and not go out for the whole weekend except for half an hour's shopping. He sat doing nothing at home. After tranquillisers proved useless, his doctor referred him to a psychiatrist.

Most people find it hard to detect, in themselves, the signs of approaching breakdown. Fiona Hulland, from MIND's Advice and Information Service, says, 'I have had men phone me up from a payphone, weeping, who are still trying to hold down their job, and talk about their state in terms of not being able to concentrate. They feel their ability to do their job is slipping and they are incredibly concerned about that. They say they can't tell their doctor about their problems, but that they need help to sort out what is happening to their life.'

Relatives, partners, flatmates and colleagues – as the above experiences show – are aware of any alteration in behaviour. A colleague at work, for example, will notice out-of-character changes: unpunctuality, a person drinking too much at lunch time, an inability to stop working, difficulty in relationships in the office. Someone living in the same house will notice obsessive behaviour worsening, or less and less food being eaten. A relative will notice a gradual withdrawal from reality.

WAYS OF HELPING

If a person is suffering from the more serious forms of mental disturbance – like hallucinations, losing touch with reality, extreme paranoia, the hearing of voices – psychiatric help is required. But sometimes in the case of people who are not functioning, are unable to cope any longer, or are very depressed, it is possible for laymen to help them.

Sometimes an outsider will see that a person is fighting a losing battle against stress, and can warn him of this. Practical help can be important here – like talking over office decisions with a colleague, or helping a post-natally depressed mother with the washing up or cleaning.

Many people are not only unable to speak to their doctor about how they feel; they cannot confide in anyone. Because they disguise or deny their feelings, it is hard to know how to help. To ask someone who is obviously depressed, for example, or becoming obsessive, if there is anything you can do to help, is asking to be snubbed. Yet it is important that people persevere in offering help, particularly as far as just listening is concerned. Fiona Hulland of MIND says, 'If you have spoken for half an hour to someone who is very depressed, and you feel you have not given them any help, they invariably say, "It's been wonderful to talk to someone about it." They sometimes say, "Do you often speak to people who feel like me?" And just to say that you do is so important. They need reassurance – particularly those who have never had anything to do with the mental health services. They may not act on what you suggest they should do, or where they should go next, but it at least makes them feel that someone cares – particularly if a person is very depressed and disillusioned and feels that no one is going to help them, and nothing will ever budge their feeling of gloom and blackness. Many phone in when they are at their lowest ebb. Listening services are very important.'

The same point was made by a Samaritan, although he stressed that a person who is seriously depressed is going to need medication. 'But that isn't enough: they are going to need support, and a lot of people are quite capable of giving it. Friends or neighbours are much more valuable than they themselves realise. The emotional rapport they may generate is very helpful, even if the other person doesn't say so. An ordinary person can befriend and support someone. The very fact that he is showing an interest and concern is of help. Afterwards, the person doesn't feel so isolated: it's a shared burden. Depressed people get lonely. At the same time, they give the impression they don't want a friend; but they do.'

Another Samaritan helper pointed out that if a person is depressed, he is probably not going to be aggressive, but may look at you vacantly. 'I would say, "I don't want to interfere, but you are looking as if you have more than the blues. If that's the case, and if you think I can help, you know where I am." That will not go unforgotten. The person may go straight past you, but he won't forget.'

Many people, especially teenagers, will back away from admitting what the real problem is. But if you can build up some sort of trust with them the real problems will emerge. It is easy to make wrong assumptions, but that only causes people to feel more alienated, because they are not communicating. They have to set the pace. Your tone of voice can give someone confidence to go on.

One problem here is that reassurance may be seen by the person concerned as a sign that you do not believe, or take seriously, the distress they feel. Often an acknowledgement of the distress will help the person accept your help ('I can see that you are very distressed and worried' or 'That must be very distressing'). Although it is reassuring to feel that someone is able to acknowledge this distress, however, to say you 'know' or 'understand' how the person feels is false. It minimises a person's experience of his problem.

'From experience,' said another Samaritan, 'the thing that people really value is not your talking, not your words, but that you are inside their skin, absolutely along with them. It makes them feel less cut off. I am surprised how some people can keep up a front. It's quite scarey because, if they break through that reserve, it's like a dam going. Yet most people do break down. It can be that they are depressed in anticipation of what might happen.'

It can be helpful to explain to people who are in a state of anxiety that the way they feel is a reaction to stress and not a sign of madness. The panic attacks that stress causes are alarming (*see Chapter 4 on anxiety and stress*), in that the physical sensations that result – like palpitations, dizziness, fainting, pounding heart – make people believe that they are having, say, a heart attack.

It can also help people ultimately if they can be brought to realise that some of their reactions are related to the past, and they may be sticking to a pattern of behaviour – like always getting involved with violent men. Or it may be that the situation they are in – perhaps living with overprotective parents – is causing suppressed resentment, which is likely to emerge as overwhelming anger in the guise of a breakdown. Quite often the person may need help to clarify what he feels about himself or his situation. But even if an outsider can see this situation clearly, and thinks that all that is needed is to persuade the person to alter his lifestyle, that person may not want to make a fundamental change in his situation.

THE EFFECT OF STRESS ON THE CARERS

Sometimes, there are two casualties: the person who has the original breakdown, and the one who cares for that person, who in turn breaks down because of the stress. It is important that the effect of this stress is realised in time, and that support – through groups of similarly placed carers – is organised. Being able to talk to people in a similar situation, who really understand what one is going through is a great help.

Many of those looking after disturbed relatives or marital partners are under enormous pressure, as is evident by the number of letters MIND receives on the subject, asking for help. One woman, for example, wrote: 'My mother, in her late eighties, has a chronic and long-standing persecution complex. She has a very suspicious nature and is convinced everyone is trying to get the better of her. Neither reasoning nor argument has any effect.'

Another woman was worried about her husband, who suffered attacks of depression lasting some three months and was only able to keep going through the help of drugs. 'I manage to cope with his tears, feelings of letting everyone down, conviction that his business is failing, his silence and not wanting to do anything, but I now find he is becoming aggressive towards me. . . . I am finding this whole situation increasingly difficult. If only I knew how other people handle the tormented outpourings when they are at their worst, or could share the feelings of loneliness, it would help.'

Another woman admitted that she was becoming disturbed at her own reactions to her husband's personality problems: 'I am beginning to suspect I am mentally sick myself and need help.'

Equally, when the crisis has passed, the patient's recovery may depend on the support of his family. If the family has allowed itself to be rendered helpless, it will clearly not be in a position to provide the help and support that the person needs. As G. K. Chesterton once said, 'We are in a very small boat in a very rough sea, and owe one another a terrible loyalty.' That loyalty may require the patient's family to make painful decisions in the interests of the family as a whole, as well as of the individual.

Ron Lacey, MIND's social work advisor, points out: 'If an individual member of the family is behaving in such a manner as to put the whole family at risk, the family may, in its own interest, have to get them out of the home. If a patient recovers, and has smashed up his own family, he has no one to come back to. And although some families cope with someone who is behaving in an impossible way, it may only be delaying the crisis to a later date. If an elderly couple are caring for a thirty-year-old son whose behaviour is intolerable, what is going to happen to him when they die?'

PRACTICAL MEASURES

Those who are on the verge of mental breakdown are not in a state to check out facilities. They, their relatives, or others concerned about them may not know how or where to get help, what amenities are available, and which organisations they can go to for assistance. MIND's Advice and Information Service will help here: it currently gets over 7,000 inquiries annually. Some of the questions most often asked are:

What do you do if you suspect the onset of mental disturbance?
The first move must be to go to a doctor, who is in a position to advise whether the symptoms are serious. The doctor can also be asked about any other facilities available – like counselling or psychotherapy. He can make a referral to the social services department for their help – if you contact them first, they will probably ask if the person has seen a doctor.

If you are contacting the doctor on someone else's behalf, the doctor will, at some point, have to see the patient: he cannot treat someone through an intermediary. Explain the circumstances and the symptoms to the doctor and ask if he will visit the person concerned. However, do not be surprised or offended if the doctor does not discuss the patient with you. While a good doctor will be concerned about his patient's difficulties, he is bound by his professional ethics not to breach the confidentiality of the doctor–patient relationship.

Supposing the person refuses to see a doctor?
This is a frequent problem. A formal visit to a doctor, or to a psychiatrist at a hospital, can frighten people and reinforce their fear that they may become 'a mental patient'. Many of those who are mentally disturbed also have no insight into their condition and refuse to accept that they are ill and need treatment. One solution is to ask, through the social services department, for a social worker to call at the house when the person concerned is there. The social worker can then generally assess the state of the person, without provoking the kind of antagonistic feelings that might occur when being seen by a medical practitioner or in a medical setting.

What services do the local health authorities provide for the mentally ill?
Details of these services can be obtained from the local social services department. Social workers are available for home visits, both to support relatives, give them practical hints on management, and discuss their difficulties and also to help the patient by listening to his problems and helping him to cope.

Patients who have left hospital, as well as those who have not required hospital treatment, may still need practical help to manage in the community. Again, the social services department can give information about day centres, workshops, clubs and residential accommodation. These services can help people readjust after being cut off from community life.

Supposing the condition worsens, and the person concerned becomes violent, or obviously in need of emergency help?
The first step again is to contact the doctor, who may suggest that the patient be admitted to a psychiatric hospital. (This requires referral by a doctor or psychiatrist.) Preferably, the patient should be admitted informally – that is, with his consent and co-operation. It is most important that the patient is given a straightforward explanation of why he would be better off with hospital treatment, and told the likely length of his stay. Patients with mental disorders are often suspicious of other people, and may believe there is a conspiracy to get rid of them; or they may sink deeper into depression.

If it is impossible to get the patient's consent to admission, the doctor may apply for compulsory admission under the terms of the Mental Health Act, 1959. (*For further information, see Chapter 9 on patients' rights.*)

There are also a few crisis centres in operation – some based in hospitals, some outside. Members of the crisis team will try to help the person over his immediate crisis, without his having to be admitted to hospital. Your doctor, or Citizens' Advice Bureau, can tell you if there is such a local service; as yet, however, there are still comparatively few.

What happens if a person needs emergency treatment when away from his doctor?

The local general practitioner will have to be called in instead, and any required admission as an in-patient will have to be in a hospital in the area where the patient is staying.

Supposing the person refuses treatment?

This is a very difficult situation, as there is no other way to insist on treatment than compulsory hospital admission. Often the only thing to be done is to keep in touch with the doctor or social worker, so that they can monitor the situation.

In law, a person may be compulsorily admitted to a hospital only if their behaviour, arising out of a mental disorder, constitutes a serious threat to the safety of the person concerned, or to other people. Often a mentally ill person's behaviour will be extremely trying. Ron Lacey of MIND gives an example of this: 'I once visited an old lady in a block of flats at the request of the housing department. This lady was in the habit of banging on the radiators for hours on end with a tin mug late at night. Understandably, this caused her neighbours considerable irritation and distress. The old lady, who was diabetic, refused the medication prescribed by her psychiatrist. However, she did take insulin injections from the district nurse. The psychiatrist, the doctor and I all agreed that it would therefore be improper compulsorily to admit her to hospital as her behaviour, although constituting a grave nuisance, was not in any way dangerous to anyone.'

What alternative treatment is there to drugs?

Find out – through your doctor, social services department, Citizens' Advice Bureau, or MIND's information service – about the nearest informal help, such as counselling services, family therapy, or a walk-in consultation centre. Some hospitals have adolescent units which carry out crisis intervention work with adolescents and their family in the community.

Sometimes stress, or emotional problems which are building up and can lead, for instance, to severe withdrawal or anxiety attacks, can be talked over with a counsellor before they become incapacitating. Some doctors work as a team with a counsellor, or the Citizens' Advice Bureau or the British Association of Counselling can give the name of the nearest counsellor. There are certain other counselling services, like the Family Service Units, which offer counselling from qualified social workers.

You can also ask your doctor to refer you to a psychotherapist if you need help in understanding and resolving the underlying problems to your emotional state. Psychotherapy, in some form, is available on the National Health Service. In the case of private treatment, the cost should be checked before embarking on any long-term commitment. It is better to contact a psychotherapist recommended by a doctor, or an organisation like the British Association of Psychotherapists, as there is as yet no official register of approved psychotherapists.

Are there any support groups for relatives?

Some of MIND's local associations act as support groups for relatives who need practical advice and a chance to exchange information with others in the same situation. The National Schizophrenic Fellowship does likewise; and some hospitals and private organisations have formed similar groups.

What about possible side-effects of drugs?

These should be checked out carefully with your doctor or psychiatrist, as well as how long after drug treatment has begun side-effects are likely to appear. MIND has published a guide to these and further details are given in Appendix I.

Supposing the doctor will not refer the person to a specialist or to a psychiatric hospital?

If a doctor is unprepared to make such a referral and will not provide satisfactory reasons for not doing so, consider changing to another doctor. This is not easy, but the Patients' Association will help over any problems of registration. If the problem deteriorates rapidly in these circumstances, go to the casualty department of the local hospital.

If there is serious disagreement with the psychiatrist's diagnosis, can anything be done?

You are entitled to a second opinion under the National Health Service, so you could seek a diagnosis from another psychiatrist by asking your doctor to refer you to one.

2

Medical Help

THE ROLE OF THE DOCTOR

Going to the doctor is the first step for those who feel that they are becoming mentally disturbed. They may be over-anxious, depressed, overexcited, not eating, or may feel persecuted. Whatever their state of mind, they are frightened: they feel matters are slipping out of their control and that they need medical assistance or treatment if they are to manage.

Admitting to a state of mental stress or disorder is not an easy thing to do. It is easier and more acceptable to claim headaches or pain than to admit to feelings of despair or persecution or to hallucinations. The doctor's evaluation here is important, as there is a genuine overlap between physical and mental illness. (Some 30 per cent of patients who are referred to medical, surgical and gynaecological out-patient departments have a psychological disorder as the basis of their symptoms.)

For this evaluation, the doctor needs to know your state of mind and what has led up to it. This is likely to take longer than the five minutes or so available during normal surgery, so ask if it is possible to have a special appointment.

The main criticisms levelled at doctors are that they usually write out a prescription without explaining it ('You'll find this will help you, Mrs So and So'); that they do not warn about possible side-effects of drugs; and that they can be unhelpful, even intimidating if questioned.

If any of these criticisms applies to your own doctor, try the following: take a friend or relation along for support if you tend to dry up; take a notebook with you containing the questions you want to ask; write down the answers in it, or arrange for the person with you to do so. Ask if it is necessary to take the treatment he suggests, and what will happen if you do not. With drug treatment, ask what it will do, how long it will take to work, and what side-effects there may be. Ask when or if you have to come back, and if there are any alternative treatments, such as some form of counselling. If, ultimately, you have consistently found your doctor unhelpful, change to another.

If, however, *you* are not honest with the doctor, it takes him much longer to diagnose your condition. Some of the more perceptive doctors are able to detect the onset of disturbance, however it is presented. As one young doctor, working in a health centre, said: 'Our task is to understand what the individual is saying. Someone may seem to be coming in with a respectable medical symptom, but it's really a passport to wanting to tell you something else, to giving you a message of some sort. I don't think we are ever very good at recognising our own states: it's not genuine dishonesty. One of the most important things a doctor can do is to make patients feel very relaxed: if you make it easy for them to talk, your own job is much easier. Listening is very important: one has to listen to make a diagnosis, to make an honest attempt to understand what is troubling someone.'

On the other hand, some professionals, while acknowledging the importance of listening, feel that direct questions are also important, in order to clarify the patient's situation. There may be good social or health reasons for the patient's feelings of depression – for example, inadequate diet, or inadequate sleep or rest.

A doctor will watch for early warning signs which the patient may be quite unaware that he is telegraphing. The first of these is why the appointment has been made: why, for instance, has a patient come to see the doctor four times in the last four weeks? It may seem to be about this or that, but the answer may be that things are not going right. A mother might come in to bring her child who has a runny nose, but what the doctor notices is that the 'ill' child is running around while the mother is sitting there looking extremely depressed and pale and does not stop talking for half an hour.

A pale, downcast expression may of course be habitual in a patient, and this is something else a doctor might notice – any change from what he knows to be normal. So if he remembers a woman as talkative and she is silent and very fidgety, he is alerted that something is wrong.

As well as a change of personality, a doctor might notice other early signs, like drinking or excessive tiredness. ('I never have a day without someone coming to me complaining of excessive tiredness,' said one doctor.) People either say that they can't get to sleep, or that they feel unrefreshed after they have slept. Students invariably say they have lost interest in their work.

Another early warning sign is when wives complain of their husband's drinking, or one of the partners has sex problems. Often people don't complain directly, because of natural reticence, but they often mention increasing marital difficulties when they get to know the doctor better. ('She's just not the woman she was, she's so bloody irritable,' or 'He's lost interest in the kids.')

Doctors can also be alerted by who comes with whom. Why does the wife want to come with the husband, or a mother with her 22-year-old daughter? An 'inappropriate' visit like that often gives a clue to the underlying problem. 'Well, wouldn't you be depressed if you were twenty-two and your mother was still coming to the doctor with you?' said one general practitioner.

'I think we are all unaware of the things which contribute to mental ill health,' said another doctor. 'People feel awful and may well not know why. We are not aware of the effect of complex relationships with our immediate families and of the build-up of past and future anxieties. It's quite common to have a fifty-year-old man who suddenly comes in with chest pains. He has no heart disease but, talking to him, you find he has been getting depressed over the last six months and, according to his wife, more and more irritable. And perhaps the sex life isn't as good. Then you find his father died of a heart attack and he is beginning to be preoccupied by his children leaving home. Suddenly, almost unknown to himself, this man, who was an extrovert at the golf club, is beginning to feel, "Has it all been worthwhile?" Men don't like losing potential.'

At this point, the doctor needs to work in collaboration with the patient so that the patient knows what is happening, and why, and the likely treatment. This, obviously, has an important effect on its outcome.

Another doctor told me that he watched for suspect physical signs: 'Either I know the patient well enough to know the sort that tells me any personal problem, or alternatively the pain doesn't have a pattern that fits with a known disease. Or a person will say he feels a lump in the bottom of his stomach, but you can find no lump. You might say to the patient, "I had a lump in my stomach when my mother died and this could be because you are upset. Are you upset about anything?" Many people find it difficult to keep a balance between various competing stresses, and this manifests itself as anxiety or pain lumps.'

At this stage, the doctor might decide whether to give the patient tranquillisers or antidepressants, to help him over a particular crisis, or refer him to a psychiatrist – or do nothing. One of the strengths of the doctor is that he does not have to make up his mind in one interview. If he suspects that something is wrong, even if the patient is not admitting it, he can make another appointment. Whether a doctor is quick to refer a patient to a psychiatrist depends very much on that particular doctor.

COUNSELLORS IN GENERAL PRACTICE

One health centre doctor I spoke to said that he himself considered that referring people to a psychiatric hospital three miles away was unacceptable and 'taking the easy option'. In his group practice, they have been taking three other courses of action. First, instead of calling on psychiatrists, they use counsellors. These are able to see people who are having difficulties which benefit from skilled counselling. They can also give more of their time than can a doctor in the middle of a busy surgery.

Second, with some of its cases, the practice works in close collaboration with the local hospital's department of psychiatry. This department has an interest in family therapy, and either the staff in the psychiatric unit visit the practice or a doctor from the practice visits them to discuss a case. They thereby review the case together.

Third, the practice has a community psychiatric nurse attached to it. She is frequently in the health centre and is able to discuss problems with both patients and doctors.

There are several advantages to both doctor and patient in having a counsellor available. Another doctor, who was very enthusiastic about counsellors, said that in his group practice 'We feel it's appropriate for a number of patients to get help on a more intensive basis, to be seen for an hour undisturbed. If somebody comes here and says they can't cope, that their husband is running away with the au pair and life has no meaning, I will see them first, and then pass them on to my counsellor. She is a colleague, part of our practice team. It's not a question of rejecting a patient and sending them off to the Marriage Guidance Council, but of explaining that I want them to see the counsellor. The counsellor is not a psychologist, not a professional, she's a working, caring, nice lady who doesn't have any hang-ups and doesn't use jargon. She's trained and she listens and gets people to look at themselves.

'A lot of patients are unhappy with their lives or their relationships or have unsatisfied goals and haven't made it – like the businessman who is still running one establishment when he dreams of running eight. It's more acceptable to be ill than to have a marital problem. But they may not want to take the advice you give them. They will hide from their problem by going to another doctor who will prescribe pills.

'Fifty years ago, with problems of this kind, you either kept them to yourself, went to your mum, or went to the vicar. But there's been an erosion of the family, and now we feel we know more than our mothers do.'

In fact, in their chapter on the primary health team in *New Methods of Mental Health Care*, Molly Meacher and Geoffrey March stress that 'the greatest opportunities for preventive work in the mental health field are provided within general practice'. They consider that one important development has been the growth of health centres and medical centres, which incorporate health visitors and sometimes social workers; and that another has been the increase in group practices, with a similarly supporting professional and lay staff. 'Of particular importance to patients with minor mental disorders are the less common experimental schemes which include social workers or counsellors within the team or, alternatively, bring a psychiatrist's skills to the surgery for perhaps a session or two each week.'

Analysis of a medical centre in Stockton-on-Tees showed that the second most common group of illnesses, after respiratory diseases, are psychiatric disorders. In other words, 'every twelfth time the consulting room door opens a patient enters who, whatever else may be the matter with him, is either depressed or anxious to such an extent that he will consult his doctor about it'.

In the Stockton-on-Tees practice, there has been an extensive and successful use of marriage guidance counsellors. The scheme started with only an hour or two of counselling a week, but the demand increased. Two counsellors are now working about twenty-four hours a week in the surgery counselling-rooms. Their hour-long consultations with patients range from the problems of lonely divorcees, to the sex problems of prisoners' wives, to patients contemplating a second marriage. They have also been the main support for patients with depression.

THE ROLE OF THE PSYCHOTHERAPIST

Other general practices have experimented with group therapy sessions. One such, which I visited in south London, has a counselling project and also runs therapy groups. Its atmosphere, as you walk through the door, is casual and friendly: chairs and cushions are scattered around a very large room and there is none of the formal feeling of a doctor's waiting-room. The therapy sessions are held here, out of surgery hours. Although the psychotherapist who runs these sessions works within the general practice team, his methods broadly illustrate what to expect from psychotherapy.

This particular psychotherapist said that most of his work at the practice 'is to do with people who come saying, "I feel I am going crazy" or are very depressed. It's known I work here as a psychotherapist. The doctor may give them some of his time, or tell them that I am available. People will come themselves with fear and feelings of paranoia, even with their own violence and anger. But when they get depressed, they come for help. Half of those I see say they feel depressed or can't cope.'

This psychotherapist finds that his crisis work with patients usually takes up to six weeks, or until they can cope with their feelings and make a decision. Sometimes, in the course of this, deeper frustrations or causes emerge and the person may join one of the two psychotherapy groups. One of these is co-counselling, the other rather more intense. Various problems are discussed within these groups and those present can explore their own and others' attitudes towards these. Some members are passive, become dependent on the group and take a lot of the anger. Through group reaction, members can discover what things they are doing to each other which are hurtful and negative. It helps them see themselves in relation to others: the group acts as a mirror.

The team feels strongly that it is absolutely useless saying, 'You are not coping, we will help by taking your feelings away by drugs.' That, in their experience, only worsens matters. They also look on 'craziness' as being a social definition. 'One girl', said the psychotherapist, 'wants to come off drugs but was warned by another doctor that if she did so, she would go crazy. What she is doing in the therapy group is, in effect, taking the opportunity to go crazy: looking at it and putting it away again. When she came to me, she said she felt as if the label of paranoid schizophrenic was her identity, she'd lived with it for so long. She felt it was no good people telling her "Be yourself", because she hadn't got a self to go back to.'

The psychotherapist felt that many of the patients coming to that general practice had been through similar pressures: 'There has been a point in their lives when they have had to erect a barrier to separate themselves from the world. Sometimes you stay in that alienated situation until the pressure from something else gets to you and overrides your defences. But, when you start talking to someone in this position, you go back to the pain that wasn't felt at the time the "separation" took place, and help them face it.' The practice is now helping an increasing number of patients with mental disorder.

THE ROLE OF THE PSYCHOLOGIST IN A GENERAL PRACTICE

One of the main advantages for patients in seeing a psychologist at the surgery, rather than at the hospital, is that they feel no stigma in just going into the next room to the doctor for their appointment, rather than being 'seen' going into a psychiatric unit or hospital. Another advantage is the informality. With a hospital referral, letters have to be written and the whole process takes longer.

In an exploratory move by the Psychology Department at Claybury Hospital in Essex, to build closer links with local doctors, a psychologist spends five hours a week working with a local general practice. Her aim has been to set up a crisis intervention service, offering individual therapy to those requiring it.

She sees about five patients a week, for about an hour each. Her colleague, a trainee psychologist, spends some twelve hours a week with patients. (There are two doctors in the practice and 6,300 patients.)

Out of a recent sample of 33 patients, the breakdown of their problems was: sex and marital problems, 7; anxiety states, 12; depression, 13; obsession, 1. These figures follow the national trend, as the largest number of people referred to psychologists are those with anxiety states and depression, followed by those with marital and sex problems.

One of her patients was a seventeen-year-old schoolgirl, who came to the doctor with a bead stuck down her ear. 'She put it there herself,' said the psychologist. 'She never told her parents and finally plucked up courage to go to the doctor to get it out. She did not come to discuss her emotional problems, but the doctor was alerted. As a result, he suggested she saw me. I see her every week, but she would never have come to the hospital for help: she hasn't told anyone she comes here to see me – she's scared she'll be labelled as mad.'

This underlines the point that, for most people, being referred to a psychologist or a psychiatrist means that they now accept themselves as being mentally ill. And relations and friends, on hearing of the referral, also tend to take this attitude. People are naturally afraid of this, and frequently will not go for help until they are seriously disturbed. Treatment then naturally takes longer. Early intervention, in the less traumatic surroundings of a family doctor's practice, is a far better solution.

In going to a doctor, people hope their problems will be solved by the right tablets. What the psychologists in the Essex surgery try to do is point out to people that stress is the overall trigger that has led to disturbances like phobias, feelings of unreality, being paranoid, or deluded about oneself or other people. They emphasise that if you can gain insight into the sort of stress which has brought on these disturbed feelings, and responsibility for control over yourself and your emotions, you are less likely to break down a second time. 'Taking tablets doesn't make everything all right,' said one. 'Nor does blaming the rest of the world, or another person, for everything that is wrong. It has to do with one's own attitude of mind.'

An example of this was a patient who came in with severe headaches, but was referred to the psychologists because there was no physical basis. It was found to be related to marital stress, but the woman considered it entirely her husband's fault that she was getting stressed. She would not accept her responsibility for her reaction to everything he did. She felt that headaches came from outside and hit her and she could not see that because she got angry she got headaches. Tablets might have cured these headaches, but the stress would still have been there.

Another patient, an Indian woman, had been very depressed long before her arrival in England, because of her husband's domineering, critical attitude towards her. In England, however, the husband could not get a job, so the wife became the main wage earner. With help from the psychologist, she built up her confidence and accepted herself as she was, rather than struggling to change to please her husband. She has now lost the feeling of stress, is more philosophical, and the relief has freed her from her irrational anxieties.

Many patients have been bewildered by their sudden inability to cope. 'I was fine until six months ago, and suddenly I got these symptoms,' is a typical remark. They feel that something alien has overtaken them, having believed themselves able to manage. But a trained outsider could see that their ability to cope was just an overlying blanket. Therapy helps them to see that the symptoms they have developed have not come out of the blue. This is perhaps particularly the case with men, who are brought up to cope and be independent, and who force themselves to believe that this is what they are like. They have never allowed themselves to break down emotionally; when their defences finally give way, under stress, they need therapeutic help to regain their confidence and ability to cope.

Perhaps the only disadvantage of psychologists, therapists or counsellors working with clients at a surgery is that this reinforces the idea that emotional problems and mental disturbances can be seen only in terms of illness rather than adjustment to a situation, or a development of one's ability to cope. If psychologists could attach themselves to the social services departments, for example, it would help give less impression that a client's problems are 'medical'.

In a paper given to the Mental Health Foundation in 1977, Dr G. Adams said that after taking on a mental welfare officer at his practice, 'The practice referral rate to consultant psychiatrists fell by about 75 per cent during the year and the admission rate to psychiatric hospitals fell by approximately the same proportion.' Interestingly, even after the mental welfare officer left, the low rate of referral stayed the same. This was thought to be due to the training the doctor received in the skills of the mental welfare officer, as well as the confidence he gained in dealing with patients' emotional problems.

No doctor can be forced to take on counselling or therapeutic help: many prefer to handle problems of mental disturbance themselves. But, as pointed out in the book *New Methods in Mental Health Care*, 'Many of the people who opt to become general practitioners are likely to be those with more interest and aptitude for chemistry and physiology than they have for dealing with interpersonal relationship difficulties.'

In the instances where some kind of counselling help has been used, with the doctor's co-operation, this has proved very successful. It is always sensible, before registering with a doctor, to meet him first to see if you find him sympathetic. At the same time, ask him if there is any counselling or therapeutic help available at the practice.

However mentally fit you may feel at the time, you might, later, be glad of such help.

THE ROLE OF THE PSYCHOLOGIST

Psychologists are not medically trained, so are not, therefore, in a position to prescribe or carry out physical treatment such as drugs or electroconvulsive therapy. Instead, they treat patients by means of 'psychological therapy' of one kind or another: behaviour therapy (aimed at changing a person's behaviour); individual and group therapy; psychoanalysis; hypnotherapy.

Sometimes, a doctor might refer a patient direct to a psychologist. Or he may refer the patient to a psychiatric out-patient clinic, and the consultant in charge may, in turn, refer the patient on to a psychologist. A patient is more likely to be referred to a psychologist if suffering from anxiety, fears, phobias, obsessions or the less severe depressive states that have a background of stress, relationship problems, and personal inadequacy.

What can one expect when one goes to see a psychologist? Dr Brian Wijesinghe, Principal Psychologist at Claybury Hospital, Essex, says: 'I usually begin by introducing myself and saying that, although I have a letter from your doctor, I like to get my information first-hand. I then ask the patient if he would like to tell me in his own words how he sees the problem and how he thinks I can be of help.

'Sometimes I find that a patient, when he has seen his GP, has been guarded in giving details of any psychological problems, and has emphasised the more physical aspects of his disorder. But when he comes to a clinic like ours, where he knows he is going to get a reasonable time to explain things, he will give a different presentation.

'We are beginning to find that people do not strictly conform to a particular diagnostic type. You might find that with someone who is phobic, you can also get an associated depressive component. Similarly, you might get patients who complain of depression and, when you question them, they probably have secondary phobic symptoms. When I question them, I usually ask them to rate or rank their problems; at certain times, one aspect comes to the fore more than others. How you treat them, therefore, will depend on what they see as their primary difficulty at the time. If they emphasise a phobia, or an obsessive condition, for example, then it is possible to use some sort of behaviour therapy approach. But if it is a more generalised depression, and they complain of feeling lethargic, pessimistic, with very little interest in what is going on, then it is more difficult to use a directive approach. My preferred treatment in that situation is either individual psychotherapy – supporting the patient, allowing him to talk through to the underlying reasons for his depression – or group psychotherapy. But that is a more long-term treatment: the average length of time is eighteen months to two years.

'Although we suggest the patient takes whatever treatment we think best, we are in a position to offer a choice. And patients who are sufficiently informed are beginning to ask for certain treatments.'

Clinical psychologists have been largely responsible for the development of behaviour therapy – which has had particular success in the treatment of phobias and obsessions. There are still many patients who are unsure as to exactly how different therapies are carried out. One woman, for example, with a spider phobia, thought that undergoing behaviour therapy would entail her being flung into a room full of spiders. It is important, as at the doctor's, to prepare any questions in advance and take a note of the answers. As Dr Brian Wijesinghe says, 'The more a patient is able to understand and accept the treatment, the greater the chances of it being effective.'

THE ROLE OF THE PSYCHIATRIST

'Patients who come to us', said one psychiatrist, 'seem to think that they are going to meet some sort of weirdy, who will look beyond their mask and find out all about them, and get all their hidden secrets. Whereas he is, in fact, an ordinary doctor who has been trained over the years to observe human behaviour and draw inferences from it.'

Most people with depression, and anxiety states, are coped with by general practitioners. But if the GP feels that the patient is in need of more specialised treatment, he may refer him to a psychiatrist. This would be done under the National Health Service – though patients can, if they wish, go direct to a psychiatrist privately. However, they will have to ask their doctor for the name of a reputable psychiatrist, as this information is not given out by the Royal College of Psychiatrists.

When a patient goes to a psychiatrist, the psychiatrist is trying to find out, first, what kind of person he is dealing with; and, second, what stresses this person is currently being subjected to. He will have in front of him the notes from the doctor, social worker, or whoever has referred the patient (unless it has been arranged privately). But he needs the patient's version of his state of mind, past history and any current pressures. A good psychiatrist will also see a relation, friend or employer, so that he can get a good overall picture. Only on the basis of this can he make a decision about treatment.

'When people come to see me,' says Dr Raghu Gaind, a consultant psychiatrist at Guy's Hospital, 'I must first evaluate them – that is, find out if there are any physical handicaps, like epilepsy, or a heart condition; or emotional handicaps like immaturity, inadequacy; or any social handicaps.

'My aim is to rehabilitate that person back into the community, taking these handicaps into consideration. I might decide that a particular woman, at the moment, cannot survive in the community, that she is very ill and must receive treatment; or that she needs support, such as coming into the day centre as a day patient; or that she only needs to be an out-patient, with perhaps a little behaviour therapy. Or possibly she does not need anything from a psychiatrist: she may say that it was her doctor's idea for her to come, and that she didn't want to.

'If a woman comes with depression, you have to ask whether she can cope with the rigours of life. If, for instance, she is a West Indian living in a colour-prejudiced area, with chronic ulcerative colitis, not very bright and very immature, she has every right to be depressed. None of these handicaps may be too severe individually, but collectively they are too much for her to handle. It may be that she will require support as an in-patient in hospital, because in our community, with the break-up of the extended family, such support at home may not be available.'

There are two main criticisms of psychiatrists. First is their seeming lack of care ('I tried to talk to the psychiatrist about my depression, but he wasn't interested'). There are, of course, good and bad psychiatrists; and they have good and bad days. But they have been built up in the public mind to be the ultimate healers, and if they disappoint these hopes and fail to come through with the expected cure the patient is bewildered and upset. Expectations of what the psychiatrist can achieve are often unrealistically high.

The second criticism is that psychiatrists only 'dish out drugs'. Patients with chronic or severe disorders may need these, as their mood can be stabilised or considerably improved by certain drugs. But, due to the medical training of psychiatrists, treatment by drugs naturally plays a prominent part. It is as well to realise that although psychiatrists will need to talk to you it is primarily to decide what action to take.

PSYCHIATRIC HOSPITAL

Some medical practitioners claim that the old stigma and fear of having to go to a 'mental hospital' has been lessened since the introduction of 'psychiatric units' within district general hospitals. But this is arguable. Certainly patients – particularly the elderly – are still nervous about what they may expect.

The routine in a psychiatric hospital or unit obviously varies considerably throughout Britain, according to what staff and internal facilities are available. The routine given below is based on that of a hospital in London, but it gives a broad idea of what to expect in other psychiatric hospitals.

On arrival, you are usually received by the sister in charge. You keep your own clothes, and your own nightclothes. Within a few hours of your admission, you will be seen by a junior doctor. This doctor will examine you physically, take a detailed history of your disorder, possibly order some investigation (like blood checks), and probably prescribe medication – to calm you, if agitated, or help your mood to change, or help make you sleep.

Within the next few days, the results of the investigations will have come in and the effect of drug treatment will have been observed. A conference is then held. This will consist of the senior psychiatrist (the consultant), the senior ward sister, junior nurses, junior doctor or doctors, possibly a psychologist, occupational therapist, and a social worker (if involved).

At this conference, your case is discussed, along with any personal problems which might have a bearing on your mental state. You may be asked to attend for a short time, and asked questions about how you feel. You will not have to answer any questions you prefer not to, but it gives you a chance to ask questions or discuss anything worrying you, as well as being an opportunity for the whole team to see you together. If it is a teaching hospital, medical students may also attend this conference.

After this, it is quite possible that you will not see the consultant until discharge point; but he is likely to be discussing your case with his junior doctor. It is important to realise this, and not feel discarded. If you are making satisfactory progress, you may not be called up to attend any further conferences, but would be seen by a junior doctor from time to time, depending on your progress. He will get reports from the nurses every day.

During the day, there is some kind of occupational therapy available – such as painting, woodwork or cooking. There may also be group therapy sessions.

Many patients complain about lack of attention ('Medical staff come and go like the elusive butterfly, and nurses say, "Catch him in the corridor if you want to speak to him" '). In a depressed or paranoid state, it is hard to realise that doctors and nurses are not avoiding you but that, again, the NHS psychiatric service is so stretched, with far too few staff, that there is not enough time to spare for many individual sessions.

When it is thought that you have recovered sufficiently to leave hospital, you will then see the consultant who will discharge you. At this point, any relevant social worker will be informed. Some psychiatric hospitals or units have a community nurse team, who can be contacted for help in any future emergency.

3

Schizophrenia

'Life with her at home continuously is a nightmare. Simple things like getting up in the morning, washing, getting dressed, going to bed without disturbing others in the house – one cannot assume any of these will happen. Demands for food and attention are insatiable. She veers from total silence at times to talking non-stop for literally hours and days and nights at a time, sometimes muttering under her breath, sometimes at the top of her voice. She raids tins and cupboards for food, eating up meals that have been planned, switches rapidly from one activity to another with restless speed, or is slumped in total passivity. . . . She has walked across railway lines at a station, and tried to jump out of moving cars. Driving with her is often unnerving. She is suspicious, and thinks people are plotting to steal her possessions. In fact, if she loses something (and this is frequently the case as all her things are in total chaos), the standard reaction is to say that someone has stolen it. She cannot manage her own affairs, but puts every obstacle in the way of anyone trying to help her.'

This account comes from *Living with Schizophrenia – by the Relatives* (published by the National Schizophrenic Fellowship), and it gives some idea of the severe problems which schizophrenia can cause.

Schizophrenia is an emotive word. Because of films like *The Three Faces of Eve*, many people believe, mistakenly, that schizophrenia means multiple personality (a condition which is a rare, though well-known form of hysteria). One woman, writing in *The Times*, said: 'The word "schizophrenia" is flung about today with flip facility, bobbing up in films, television scripts, literary criticism, even political articles, mostly as some sort of modish synonym for indecisiveness.

But no one who has seen the actual medical condition would ever want to use it except in its correct context.'

Schizophrenia was originally called 'dementia praecox' (early madness). It was Eugene Bleuler, in a psychiatric handbook published in 1911, who first suggested the name schizophrenia (from the Greek, meaning 'splitting of mind'). He considered this more exactly portrayed the 'splitting', distortions and disturbances which take place in a schizophrenic's thoughts, feelings and perceptions.

The onset of schizophrenia may come at any stage of life, though it is most frequently found at adolescence and early adulthood. Statistics vary, but on the whole men are a little more often affected than women; single people more than married; and those living in large cities more than those in villages.

SYMPTOMS

The symptoms of schizophrenia are disorders of thought, perception, emotion and body movement. They fall into four main categories. The first of these is known as the *simple type* and include a general deterioration of personality; difficulty in concentration; lack of depth in relationships; illogical thought; less interest in outside events; insufficient, or wrong, emotion for a certain situation. These symptoms usually set in during or after adolescence. The *hebephrenic type* includes the hearing of hallucinatory voices, which vary in clarity, but which are quite real to the person concerned. These voices are sometimes attributed to radio waves, telepathy, electronic apparatus. Delusions may occur, such as believing that announcements on the radio or television have a personal meaning. The *catatonic type* is characterised by alternating periods of unpredictable excitement and stupor. Movement is affected: some sufferers become nearly immobile or take up stilted postures. Predominant in the *paranoid type* are delusions of persecution. Voices are heard, but they are hostile; the sufferer believes he is being watched, plotted against, or persecuted by certain people, usually social, political or racial groups.

GENETIC RISK

Many parents, if there has been schizophrenia in the family, worry that this condition will be inherited by their children. Although the condition itself cannot be inherited, the predisposition towards schizophrenia is naturally higher among 'first-degree' relatives, such as children, than 'second-degree' relatives, like nephews and nieces. The child most at risk is the one whose parents are both schizophrenic. However, there is a wide area of chance here. Counsellors who can specifically advise on genetic risks are now attached to some general hospitals and family doctors can refer their patients to them for advice.

ENVIRONMENT AND FAMILY

Stressful events, or stress within the family, may play a part in bringing on symptoms of schizophrenia – as it may with any kind of mental disturbance. One of the suggested causes of schizophrenia most publicised in recent years has been the character and attitudes of the patient's family. R. D. Laing in *The Politics of Experience* says: 'Without exception, the experience and behaviour that gets labelled schizophrenic is a special strategy that a person invents in order to live in an unliveable situation.' The view here is that developing schizophrenia is a way of coping with intolerable circumstances within the family. In some instances, the family as a whole may require treatment.

Nevertheless, supporters of this view sometimes forget that it is usually the family who have to look after the person suffering from schizophrenia, and to whom the person is likely to return after treatment. To make a family feel responsible for the illness, in these circumstances, is unconstructive and may do harm.

THE EXPERIENCE OF SCHIZOPHRENIA

There have been, and still are, a great many arguments about schizophrenia, its possible causes, varying diagnoses, and even whether it exists.

No single experience is precisely like another. But, to give an idea of the illness, here is the experience of a girl in her twenties, who was diagnosed as suffering from schizophrenia a few years previously. When I saw her, at 4 p.m. one day, she still lay huddled in bed, and had to be encouraged to take her daily medication before she could concentrate.

The first signs of an alteration within herself had come when she was about twenty-one. 'I began to look at people in a different way, to study them more than I used to. I thought perhaps I was learning to be more astute and did not take much notice. At the time, my job was that of a reservations clerk. When I was taking a reservation one day, I heard a voice speaking to me. I thought, that wasn't the passenger, surely, and shook my head and carried on. But this voice kept coming back. It was saying things like, "You are Sylvia, aren't you?" And I would hear myself saying, "Yes, I am Sylvia." And then it would say, "How do you do?" It was as if someone was trying to make contact with me, trying to get me from the next world. The voices never came at home, but they came more and more at work, and I started to make a lot of mistakes. So I took a holiday abroad.'

On the journey, she began to feel as if she was floating. Although she was swimming and going out with friends, she could not talk to them or tell them how she felt. The voices continued, saying that they were such-and-such a person – she could never quite catch the name. The strain caused her to cry constantly and she finally returned home. She could hardly speak without stuttering at that point, and the things people said to her made no sense.

She went to the doctor, who prescribed drugs which would clear her mind and make her more active, as she was getting very lethargic. These helped, but made her feel very restless: she would go out in the middle of the night and not return until early morning. She became irresponsible and did not want to go back to work. 'I still heard the voices,' she said. 'They said things like "You are very nice" and would describe some of the nice things about me. But then one particular voice started to goad me, to say things like "You can't do that if I say you can't" and "You must obey me" and "If you don't obey me you will be sorry." In the end I cut my wrist to prove to it that if I wanted to do anything at all, I could.'

After that, she was admitted to psychiatric hospital for observation and ended by staying there for nine months. On admission, she explained that she thought the voice was that of Tutankhamun and that his curse was on her. Her main reason for thinking this was that the voice told her that she would die young, just as he had. 'I had a record of a song called "All the gods die young" and I used to play it, and the two words "Die Young" used to stand out, as if emphasised for me to hear.'

She enjoyed her stay in the psychiatric ward, because the other patients in the ward were sympathetic: they, too, had voices that told them to harm themselves. She took the medication given to her, but heard her voices constantly. They often told her to go home, and she would do so, and be persuaded by her family to return. Through losing her temper with the voices, which kept telling her to do things such as going into other people's beds, or saying that she would die in a few years' time, she would sometimes become violent and smash a window, and need sedation.

While in hospital, she went to group therapy every morning and saw her doctor there every two weeks. 'He would ask me if I had known anything about Tutankhamun or Egyptology. But, if it was Tutankhamun's curse, I couldn't understand why he should pick on *me*.'

Despite medication, her thoughts remained chaotic. 'The madness is like a noise, the whole time in your head,' she said. 'People are talking to you and you can't understand what they are saying and your head is exploding with this kind of rubbish and dreams and things that can't be expressed. I think it's a life struggle, my struggle. It manifests itself as a kind of permanent scream. But I hear birds singing sometimes very clearly: that stays in your mind. So do the expressions people have on their faces, if they are shouting to their kid or saying, Come here quick. Your eyes seem wide open, but you never quite know where you are.'

The hospital discharged her at that stage, as her bed was needed and she seemed reasonably stable. She stayed at home a year, then became confused again – writing notes to herself, waking her family up at night, staying out. The voices still pestered her, although they were less taunting. She returned to hospital and was put on a different medication, which seemed to be quite successful. After several months she went home, and continued with group therapy, and occupations like pottery, at a day centre. Unable to maintain interest, she left. She remains on medication, but since then she has stayed at home.

'The main thing about schizophrenia', she said, 'is stagnancy: everything slows down, like a record when you turn the speed down. In the three or four years since it began, I've just fluctuated. I've gone through stages when I have not known what is happening within me and I've just had to tuck myself up in bed. Everything goes blank, like sliding down a chute into deep water. My blank days and moments now only come every six months or so and I think it's because I am more content and have more peace of mind. I don't hear the voices so much now, though they will sometimes still urge me to do things like make a cup of coffee, have a bath or wash my face. It doesn't come from me, but from Tutankhamun. I get my medication every fortnight, but because of the tablets I take it takes me ages to wake up and I have no incentive to get me going.' She wrote a note to herself, then screwed it up. It read 'I know where I'm going, but I'm not going there.'

RELATIVES

This girl – although existing rather than living – was at least more stable and manageable on her medication. But the strain on her family was considerable – getting her to take the pills, preventing restless wandering at night, encouraging her not to stay in bed all day.

The puzzling nature of schizophrenia is as distressing to the partner or relatives as to the patient – unsure, as they are, whether there will be one or more episodes of the illness, how acute these will be, or whether it will become chronic. The behaviour of the schizophrenic is also bewildering, upsetting and frightening – as is any change of personality in someone you know well. One woman, worrying about her son who had been diagnosed schizophrenic some five years previously, said she did not know how to cope: 'His condition is giving me cause for alarm and despondency the last few weeks. He has developed a marked persecution syndrome, citing a particular person whom he avers reads his mind and communicates by telepathy. He appears completely incapable of controlling his own life.'

Another man said, of his daughter: 'The strain of looking after her is very great as my wife and I are pensioners. She will sit in my flat giving vent to whirling, confused speech, blinking rapidly and with spasmodic jerking of legs and hands. After about five minutes she calms down. All the floor space and much of the furniture is covered with carrier bags containing assorted rubbish, some taken from dustbins. She now takes with her, everywhere, several carrier bags filled with all manner of useless objects and a very heavy handbag, similarly full.'

A sister of a schizophrenic woman, who was in her early forties and lived at home, also spoke of the misery it caused her parents. Her sister had no steady job, and at night would cry and bang her head against the wall.

Another couple were equally distressed about their schizophrenic son of twenty-three, who had been in and out of hospital since the age of sixteen: 'He comes home from hospital improved, but has no job, no purpose in life, no friends. He spends most of his time in his room, playing records. Sometimes he draws and paints, but soon gets lonely and depressed. He exists in a sort of limbo between relapses and hospital treatment.'

Many other parents felt, in a way, that their child had never grown up, that they still had to take the full burden of responsibility for them: 'Since he left school, he has found it increasingly difficult to adjust to adult life or to hold down a job or to concentrate his thoughts or act responsibly.'

Many relatives emphasised the complete disruption a schizophrenic can cause: to have to listen, for example, as one parent did, night after night, to violent sobbing, hysterical laughter, obscene abuse; and, in the daytime, watch her daughter stay crouching under a blanket, afraid of everything. The burden of caring for the schizophrenic so often falls on the family. One father said that he did not know what to do about his thirty-year-old daughter, who had been sent home from hospital. 'She was treated for schizophrenia at the hospital, but finally the doctor maintained he could do no more for her, as she would not co-operate with the hospital and was impossible to control.'

Another woman said: 'We have a son with severe schizophrenia, but as you know they are all for getting psychiatric patients back into the community. Our son is one of the family now, but what happens to him when anything happens to us?' As nine out of ten patients in psychiatric beds in hospital now remain in-patients for less than a year – and in Britain some 80 per cent of patients under sixty-five who have been continuously in hospital are diagnosed schizophrenic – this problem of caring for them is on the increase.

Research by the National Schizophrenia Fellowship, reported in their booklet *Schizophrenia at Home*, shows that relatives at home needed help and advice in the following areas:

INITIAL INFORMATION

Many families simply do not know what is happening when a person in that family starts behaving strangely – talking in a bizarre way, relating strange events which are claimed to have happened. Even if they have heard of the word 'schizophrenia', they may not understand what it can entail.

The first step is to contact the doctor, who will assess the person's condition and probably refer him for psychiatric treatment. (You could, of course, go direct to a psychiatrist, privately, if you prefer.) Sometimes a schizophrenic will not admit he is ill, so you may have to make the initial visit to the doctor on your own, and get his advice and try to arrange for him to call. After he has seen and assessed the person, ask what the diagnosis is, and what it means in practical terms. (Will he have to go into hospital? Is he likely to harm himself or others? What should you do if his behaviour suddenly worsens?) It may be too early to assess the likely outcome, but nevertheless ask about this.

If the doctor believes it to be schizophrenia, one way of finding out more about the illness is to contact the National Schizophrenic Fellowship, which issues a great deal of explanatory material about schizophrenia and, specifically, the problems which relations may encounter.

CONTACT WITH SERVICES

Many relations do not know what, or whether, there are any other services that can offer practical help.

An approach can be made through the local social services department for a social worker to visit the family. There is, however, a serious lack of counselling services. The National Schizophrenia Fellowship runs various groups, which give an opportunity to exchange information and experiences with others who either care for schizophrenics or have been schizophrenics themselves. Some local associations of MIND can also be of help in this connection.

MEDICATION

The problems here were that relatives did not know how to ensure that a patient took his medication after discharge from hospital. Some did not see the importance of medication. Others were worried about side-effects.

It may be possible to get a community psychiatric nurse to visit the patient regularly to administer an injection. Or if the injection is normally given by a doctor, and the patient fails to turn up, the doctor could be asked to pay a home visit. Regular medication is extremely important in stabilising the mood of the schizophrenic, although this often means time spent in persuading the patient to take tablets. Problems in this area should be immediately referred to the doctor or psychiatrist. There are side-effects to the required drugs – which may well contribute to the patient's reluctance to take them. Ask the medical practitioner exactly what to expect.

HOSPITAL AFTERCARE

Relatives found they needed more information about the problem of living with a schizophrenic after he returned home from hospital.

They did not know what behaviour to expect, or what to do about it.

Some hospitals have a community psychiatric nurse service. If this is the case, ask for one who has seen the patient in hospital to visit. This can be of great support to both the ex-patient and family. Similarly, try to arrange for a social worker to visit the home routinely after discharge. You will need all the support you can get. The family doctor should have been advised of the general condition of the patient after discharge, in case any emergency arises, but visit him to make sure of this and to ask if he has any suggestions or advice to give. Sleeplessness may also put a strain on the marriage. Patients also respond better to consistent firmness and a certain amount of structure in their lives. An outside person with some authority – such as a psychiatric nurse – can be helpful here, particularly over taking medication.

TREATMENT

In the last twenty years, new drugs have been very effective in treating schizophrenics. They can control hallucinatory voices, calm excitement and diminish severe disorders of thought and delusions. They also help make the schizophrenic's behaviour less antisocial and lessen withdrawal from ordinary life.

These drugs can be taken daily in tablet form or they can be injected, at longer intervals. The importance of maintaining the schizophrenic on them is stressed by Dr Raghu Gaind, a consultant psychiatrist at Guy's Hospital. He checked on 111 schizophrenic patients, and found that only thirteen were taking their tablets. 'This is quite understandable,' said Dr Gaind. 'As soon as they felt better, through the pills, they stopped. Those suffering from schizophrenia have little insight: they do not consider themselves to be ill. And the side-effects can be unpleasant. So they stop.' Eighty patients, maintained on drugs for two years, remained symptom-free. Half of these were then kept on drugs and, during the following year, only one patient relapsed. The other half were given placebos (non-active tablets) and nearly three-quarters of them relapsed within nine months.

Drugs also help patients to cope with upsetting events, which have been found to trigger off episodes of schizophrenia. In that case, as the drugs are strong, would it not be better to administer them only at times when those concerned need particular support? 'Once a patient has gone off drugs, it is hard to get him on again,' says Dr Gaind. 'Once they feel better physically through not being on drugs, they do not want to restart them. But what may be possible, instead of giving them large doses all the time, is to maintain them on small doses and raise these when particular support is needed.'

It is important to be aware that upsetting events can worsen a schizophrenic's behaviour and mood and that extra support of some kind may be needed. The schizophrenic may have to be helped to lead a rather narrow life between understimulation and over-stimulation.

PSYCHOTHERAPY

Psychotherapy is rarely used in schizophrenia because of the acute difficulties imposed by the patient's lack of insight. Also, there is a risk that the patient's condition may be aggravated by it. However, psychotherapy may often be given in conjunction with certain drug treatment.

DAY HELP

If those who have to care for the patient after discharge are at work during the day, the social services department can help to arrange for attendance at a day centre, or for admission to a hostel. An ex-patient can live in a hostel independently, which may help relations to cope by allowing them an extended break from caring. In some cases, he or she may need sheltered environment for the rest of his life. The social services department can advise here.

If the person concerned is able to enter into any occupation during the day, it could stop any deterioration in his condition. A job is the best answer, but this may not be practical. Those with schizophrenia often encounter problems at work, as they tend to be hypersensitive to criticism and are also frequently frustrated because of having to do a job below their capabilities. The Disablement Resettlement Officer will also have information on industrial rehabilitation units, where those who have been out of work are assessed and suitable training recommended. One advance warning here is that there is not automatically a job available at the end of the training.

Should a job be out of the question, a social worker will be able to arrange for the person concerned to attend a nearby day centre. Activities at any centre vary, but there are a variety of occupations like woodwork or painting.

FINANCIAL SUPPORT

Sickness benefit can be obtained by getting a three-monthly sickness certificate from the doctor. If a person starts a job, and then has to give it up through being too ill to manage, he will have to reapply for sick pay. More detailed information can be obtained from the *Disability Rights Handbook*.

PRACTICAL SUGGESTIONS

1 If you have any worries about the behaviour of a member of the family, discuss these with your doctor. It may be that you have no need to worry; but if there is a possibility of schizophrenia, the earlier medical attention is received, the better.

If the doctor tells you that he does not think there is anything to worry about, and, if after a time, you feel there is further deterioration, go back and say so and, if necessary, ask for a referral to a psychiatrist. Be honest about the situation. Do not just say that you are still a little worried about your relation's health: tell the truth – which is usually that you cannot stand it any longer.

2 The burden of caring for the person – who may not go into hospital, or who will go in but then return – falls heavily upon the family. Partners and family members can soon become exhausted by their day-and-night restlessness. It is better, as the carer, not simply to stay at home and 'watch', but to take a job, or get out of the house

as often as possible. Otherwise there is a danger of getting interwoven with, or exacerbating, the illness of the person who is at home, and not keeping a separate identity. If the person is not well enough to be left at home, in case he damages it, or harms himself, he should really be in hospital.

Sometimes an annual rest for the carer is an urgent requirement, and in these circumstances it is sometimes possible to arrange for the patient to be looked after for a short period, either in or outside hospital. This can be done through the social services department, or contact the National Schizophrenic Fellowship for advice.

3   The importance of support groups as a way of getting practical advice and sharing the problems of caring cannot be overemphasised. This reduces tension and members can arrange telephone links between each other, to help in an emergency. Information about these relative support groups, as well as social and family after-care for patients, can be obtained from the National Schizophrenic Fellowship. This is a national organisation concerned with all matters to do with the relief of sufferers from schizophrenia and the problems of their families. Meetings organised by the local associations of MIND can also act as a support to relatives and schizophrenic sufferers.

4   Remember that some people suffer from one attack of schizophrenia and then remain perfectly healthy for the rest of their lives.

5   If the sufferer has to take medication, ask the medical practitioner for exact details about when, and how many, tablets must be taken. Ask whether the more long-term injections would be possible. Ask for particulars of any likely side-effects, so that these do not take you by surprise.

6   Some chronic sufferers may need long-term supervised accommodation for the rest of their lives. But sometimes they need only go to hospital for two or three weeks while their medical balance is worked out and the correct medication prescribed. Some 10 per cent of people may have only one schizophrenic attack.

7   Check whether there are any social facilities for ex-patients run by the hospital. One social worker, based in a teaching hospital, holds a weekly evening club. Some 60 to 70 per cent of those attending have schizophrenia and it shows them that they can take part in

normal, social life, with activities like drama, and discos. They can often dance their way into a calmer frame of mind. If they are finding their voices particularly bothersome, it is suggested for their sake that they go home. The social worker herself says, 'What people do not do enough of is put an arm around them when they are distressed or frightened. Even if they are as stiff as ramrods, they relax after a time and feel comforted.'

8 Those who want more detailed information about schizophrenia, its symptoms, causes, care provision and so on, can contact the National Schizophrenia Fellowship, which has a wide publication list. The Office of Health Economics has also published a booklet called *Schizophrenia?*

4
Anxiety and Stress

'I was sitting in a chair one night,' said a young man, 'when all of a sudden my legs went weak and a feeling of tension seemed to pass up my body to my head, causing me to get into a severe state of panic and fear. I was very shaky all night long: from that day onwards, I have lived in a permanent state of tension and tiredness. I have been in a mental hospital for anxiety depression, which is what the doctors say I have. I live each day with severe exhaustion. I have been told to "cure myself" and "pull myself together", but when your head is tense every day of your life, what can you do? Because I cannot concentrate, I cannot hold a job. I honestly feel one day my brain will just explode and I will be left a mental cabbage.'

Anxiety states rank second to depression as the most common psychiatric disorder. Anxiety itself is a normal, indeed useful feeling, as it alerts people to trouble, or motivates them into dealing with it. It is also an understandable reaction to stressful events or an unacknowledged internal conflict. It can, of course, be a symptom of another underlying disorder, such as a physical disease.

There are two main categories of anxiety: *generalised anxiety* (resulting in anxiety or panic 'attacks') and *phobic anxiety* (a response of intense fear and panic to a *specific* object or situation).

ANXIETY OR PANIC ATTACKS

What is frightening about these anxiety or panic attacks is that the violent sensations they bring convince the sufferer that he is physically ill, perhaps having a heart attack. They can include palpitations, rapid heartbeat, pain in the chest, dizziness, faintness, breathing difficulty, choking, weakness in the legs, nervous shaking, feelings of panic and loss of control, fear of dying. This is because the body goes on 'red alert' when faced with a threat. Extra blood is diverted to the muscles of the arms and legs, in case of 'flight or fight.' As this blood is diverted from organs like the stomach and intestines, the result is unpleasant sinking feelings or weakness.

Intermittent attacks of anxiety, which are the feature of *generalised anxiety*, come without warning (as with the example which begins this chapter). They are not necessarily tied up with any upsetting event, but perhaps a general build-up of stress which may have gone unnoticed. Because of this, the person concerned naturally imagines he is physically ill, and will go to the doctor. The doctor, in turn, checks him out physically, possibly arranging a further investigation at a hospital. When his physical condition, including heart, is confirmed in good order, the 'patient' is satisfied that it was a single incident. Then, again without warning, he has another attack. These might start to fall into a pattern of every few months, days or even minutes. The severity of the sensations might fluctuate. But they may be troublesome enough to make the person irritable, upset, nervous, frightened, even confined to bed.

It is hard to realise, or accept, that such intense physical sensations can be caused by mental stress – either a slow build-up over the years or a sudden traumatic event. We keep the mental and physical side of our lives in separate compartments: it is important to realise the effect one can have on the other. It is equally important to realise that, however well you may think you are coping, long-term stress and strain – such as a demanding job, a demanding spouse, a constantly crying child – finally has its effect.

One woman in her early thirties, for example, experienced such a severe anxiety attack that she thought she was going mad. 'I was lying awake one night,' she said, 'feeling rather depressed, thinking of various things that had gone wrong. Suddenly I had this great clanging noise in my head; my heart was thumping and my head reeling with waves of dizziness.' She underwent various hospital tests, as she was convinced she had a brain tumour. Only when she realised that she was physically all right did she accept that it could be due to the pressures she was facing.

A year earlier she had moved to a different job in an airline reservations department, where she never sat next to the same person two days running, and formed the habit of not talking much to colleagues. This led to her gradually becoming withdrawn, particularly as the man she was living with worked late at nights, and she was often alone. Her expressed belief that he was working harder than he need, and deliberately coming home late, strained their relationship. She also felt that she was at a critical age – thirty-two – and was afraid that she might regret not having children. She worried over whether she should marry the man she lived with, and whether her career was successful enough. A few months previously, her hearing-aid had been stolen, and she could not afford to replace it. Having longed to buy a house, she and her partner were now doing so and the commitment this entailed only added to her feelings of stress. She began to suffer from hypochondria and became scared that her drinking and smoking was affecting her health. The scene was set for the kind of anxiety attack that she suffered.

After she was found to be physically well, her doctor prescribed tranquillisers. When she found that these were not calming her sufficiently, the doctor suggested stronger drugs. But the side-effects of these worried her and she stopped. 'Just getting reassurance from anybody is the greatest help I can have,' she said. 'With that help, I think I can get through – as long as I can convince myself that there is really nothing physically wrong with me and that I'm just being neurotic.'

Anxiety attacks often occur after the stress of a change of job, job promotion, or even an additional job. One man, for example, who had agreed to help out a friend who was running a pub, said that he brought some sandwiches up to the bar, but 'as I approached the customers, I suddenly felt panic. My heart beat very fast, I had excessive sweating and violent shaking in both hands. One of the customers told me not to worry about it, and I got over it.' However, other panic attacks followed and he decided to move to a different area. The attacks continued, even though the new job went well, but as they were not evident to anyone but himself, he felt he could cope.

The severity of anxiety attacks often results in people leaving their jobs. 'I'm terrified of sitting at a meeting,' said one woman, 'in case I should collapse and die of a heart attack.' And a nineteen-year-old said she had 'recently had to leave my job as a secretary because of trembling attacks'. A third young woman said: 'I can't seem to keep a job for long as I feel everyone is looking at me and all I want to do is run from whatever I'm doing.' She admitted that her doctor had told her she would not faint. 'But when your heart is thumping away and your head starts spinning, I honestly think that I am going to die.'

The fear of these attacks occurring again is as crippling as the actual attacks themselves. One man said: 'I'm now frightened to get up in the morning to face the next day, and I get frightened, too, at things that I used to enjoy before – like going to work, going to dances. I try to beat it by forcing myself to go.'

Another woman found that she could not wait for a bus for any length of time: 'I start walking, or do not go wherever I was going. If I go into a shop and it looks like a long wait, I walk away until I find a shop with fewer people in it.'

The experience of a severe anxiety attack at work worried one woman so much that 'I beg my husband not to leave me in the house on my own when he has finished work. Also, he has to come shopping with me, and once there I feel I can't let him out of my sight in case my fears are realised and I collapse.'

PHOBIC ANXIETY

Because these anxiety attacks can occur at any time, and in any place, it is likely that a great many will happen outside the house, in the street, say, or the supermarket. The person then fears entering that situation again, in case of experiencing another embarrassing and frightening attack. Agoraphobia – from the Greek, meaning 'fear of the market place' – is not a fear of actual open spaces, as it is often described. It is the fear of what could happen in the 'market place' – the fear, that is, of an anxiety attack in public.

The result of all this fear, and panic attacks, is that the person only feels safe inside the home: some agoraphobics have not left their house for years. They develop dependency on their partner and accept the limitations of their life.

Unfortunately, fear of one situation can easily spread to another, so a fear of going outside can extend to a fear of being on a bus or in a train or restaurant. 'I can't get across any main road to get to the shop, or go on a bus,' said one woman. 'I'm afraid to go shopping or even hang my washing up in the garden,' said another.

There are other situations which can cause anxiety and panic attacks to those who need to be totally in control at all times – being in an aeroplane, for example, or a lift, or a crowded room which they cannot easily leave.

Panic attacks also occur if a person with a fear of a specific object – such as a cat, dog, spider or snake – is suddenly faced with this object. The shock of the encounter can cause near hysterical panic: in one instance, a spider phobic attacked a colleague who had dangled a spider in front of him; in another, a wasp phobic, buzzed by a wasp, deserted her young baby and ran screaming down the street.

The cause of a person's fear of a specific object may well be rooted in a childhood incident: children take delight in locking other children into rooms, putting spiders down their friends' necks or frogs in their desk. Someone with an anxious personality may well retain their fear into adulthood. Behaviour therapy (see Appendix I) has proved reasonably successful in treating this kind of phobia.

The causes of agoraphobia and what is sometimes called 'social phobia' (fear of social situations) are more complex. But stress plays a major part. In fact, agoraphobia has sometimes been called 'the calamity syndrome' because it so often sets in after a calamity. A period of stress, causing a build-up of anxiety, culminates in a traumatic event such as an operation, or the death of a parent. The sufferer may, at the time, appear to be coping: then an anxiety attack takes place suddenly – say 3 p.m. one Tuesday afternoon, several months after the event. The person doesn't link it to recent, or past events, considers it a sign of physical illness, and fears, after another attack, to leave the house. In this way, agoraphobia is the most disabling of all the phobias.

Understanding that stress is behind the condition does not

necessarily mean that those concerned recover instantly – although it has been known – but it does at least relieve the additional secret fear that they may be physically or mentally deteriorating. This can be very incapacitating. As one woman said: 'For about six months, I have been suffering from an intense fear of mental illness. Most of my waking hours are filled with thoughts of it and even when I am very busy I always have a feeling of anxiety in the background.'

OBSESSIVE PREOCCUPATIONS AND COMPULSIVE RITUALS

Equal irrational anxiety is also felt by those people suffering from obsessive patterns of thought and behaviour. They may become obsessed with the idea, for example, that they might convey or acquire infection (so will wash themselves, or the bath, constantly). Or they may fear they could cause injury or harm (so tidy away objects or clothes over which others might trip). They fear the consequences of not carrying out these acts: if they do not do so, they believe, they will face some strange retribution, like eternal damnation or the death of a loved one.

The way of warding off this retribution is to carry out protective rituals. Their lives, because of these rituals, become extraordinarily complicated. A room may take all day to clean because it has to be done in a certain way; similarly, dressing in the morning may not be completed until the evening.

Perhaps the most usual compulsive act is constant hand-washing, often using a particular ritual. For example, one woman, who had an obsessive fear of touching an 'unclean' object, would wash her right arm from fingers to wrist, from wrist to elbow and from elbow to upper arm, and then repeat this on her left arm – and would continue to do so until her anxiety had lessened. It could be fifty times a day.

Checking rituals before going to bed at night can also take hours. All clothes might have to be checked several times to ensure that they are facing the same way, and that they have no fluff or specks caught in linings or hem.

Any attempt to prevent these rituals from being carried out can cause serious upset. Yet, properly monitored, this has proved one of the most effective treatments for this condition. Although the person's anxiety level shoots up, with relaxation and the help of a therapist it can eventually be contained and overcome. The only remaining problem is that, if you take away the activities with which the obsessive has been filling his days, something has to replace these, or depression quickly fills the gap.

STRESS AND TENSION

The reaction to stress and tension varies: instead of having anxiety attacks, a person may suddenly find himself unable to cope. One man, for example, who was setting up a window-cleaning business as well as working in a pub, became increasingly exhausted and tense after his constant 6 a.m.–11 p.m. working day. His wife was aware of this, but did not think it too serious. After six months, he suddenly broke down and cried in front of his family and could hardly speak for the next few weeks.

One nineteen-year-old girl feared that she was going out of her mind: 'I've had a bit of job stress. For about a month I have felt really strange, like I was in limbo or something, and everybody and everything seems cut off.' There is little awareness of the effect of stress, or that time is running out. 'It happened all of a sudden,' said one man in bewilderment. 'I thought I was coping very well and then I got a promotion and suddenly I was not getting to work on time, making excuses. In the end I had to leave because of my bad record of work and I went on the dole. I finally went to the doctor and got some pills and they worked for a couple of weeks. Then I knew this was no good, so I went to the hospital and had an interview there. I spent most of the time in tears because I was trying to describe my life and what went on and became incoherent. I went back as far as being evacuated.'

RELAXATION AND CONTROL OF TENSION

Meditation and yoga are ways of lowering tension, basically through the use of relaxation. And learning how to relax is obviously of great importance to those suffering from anxiety and tension. In his book,

The Art and Practice of Relaxation, Ian Martin explains how to attain full relaxation and how these techniques can be used to counter tension headaches, insomnia, fear of social situations, asthma and eczema.

His progressive series of simple relaxation exercises, which take about half an hour, start with lying down on a firm bed in a quiet, warm, dimly lit room. The next step is to make the body as tense as possible before letting all the muscles go limp. You should then, he says, make your breathing slower and deeper, before bringing a picture of any single object into your mind's eye and concentrating totally on this. Finally, imagine as realistically as possible that you are lying on a warm beach or in a country field. The effects of this regular daily exercise are calming and reduce the build-up of tension.

The use of biological feedback machines is another way of controlling tension. The basic way in which a biofeedback machine works is that it monitors and informs you of what is happening at various stress indicators in the body. For example, after registering pulse and perspiration level, it might emit a high-pitched tone which goes higher with increased tension and lower with less tension. By concentrating on the meter's signal, you can learn to lower its tone. Once this has been achieved you can, in time, learn to lower your anxiety and tension level without the use of this machine.

Physical exercises can also lower mental tension. This is particularly so with the Chinese Tai Chi exercises. These are a series of rhythmic movements, in which you use the disposition of body weight to relax the whole body.

Everyone probably has a preferred way of relaxation. What is important, however, is to keep a certain time of the day apart for this relaxation – even if it is just watching television – and to be aware of the possible effects of that job promotion, new house, relationship break-up. Unnoticed, and unattended to, they may cause you to break down; and a quick burst of relaxation exercises will be of no use at all.

SELF-HELP FOR FEARS AND ANXIETY

In his book *Living with Fear*, Isaac Marks stresses the golden rules about anxiety: that it is unpleasant, but rarely harmful; that escape from the situation or object of fear should be avoided and facing it should be encouraged; that the longer and more rapidly the worst is faced, the quicker the fear will fade. This is by no means easy for the phobic. One agoraphobic I spoke to said firmly that if she went outside she would die. Encouraged, gently, over several sessions to do so, she did get as far as the gate. She then had, as she anticipated, a severe anxiety attack – palpitations, sweating, near fainting. It was highly unpleasant; but she did not die. Instead of being helped indoors, she was encouraged to go on. She had two more anxiety attacks before reaching the end of the street; but she had at least been outside after more than six months of rigidly staying inside the house. After that breakthrough, she was able, slowly, to resume her normal life.

Isaac Marks, in his book, gives various practical remedies to alleviate anxiety. For instance, if you feel you cannot breathe deeply, he suggests you take a deep breath and hold it as long as you possibly can. In about a minute, your reflexes will force you to take another deep breath. On the other hand, if your anxiety is making you take too many deep breaths, resulting in tingling in the fingers and painful contractions of hands and feet, he suggests you hold a paper bag over your mouth. This means you inhale back the carbon dioxide just breathed out, and the overbreathing is likely to stop. An inability to swallow can be overcome, he suggests, by chewing a dry biscuit until it is moist: eventually, swallowing it will be automatic.

Some fears, like those of students who panic totally at examination time, may need the help of a college psychologist or counsellor if they are the product of anxieties about failing to live up to parents' expectations. At London University, one psychologist holds examination seminars, to teach exam phobics 'anxiety management'.

Anxiety management usually involves the use of strategies, thought about and prepared for in advance. If you know, for instance, that you are going to go for a job interview, plan on getting there early so that you do not become more anxious by being late; take deep breaths while waiting to be called in; have some questions ready to ask the interviewer; practise looking someone in the face for a short period, rather than keeping your eyes lowered. If you know you will soon be retiring, or suspect you are a candidate for redundancy, plan in advance what to do with the extra leisure time. If you anticipate feeling claustrophobic in the cinema, choose a seat near the exit. Anxiety feeds on itself: working out a positive programme of attack has the additional advantage of switching your thoughts into a different, calmer and less chaotic channel.

ASSERTIVENESS TRAINING

This technique, used perhaps more in America than in Britain, is useful in creating confidence and overcoming anxiety in those who are inherently anxious and insecure about their job, their looks, their sexual and social behaviour. Although it is often carried out with the aid of a therapist, it can be done individually.

One method is to make a private list of occasions when you have been 'non-assertive' – for example when you have accepted cold soup or coffee in a restaurant, have held in your feelings to avoid a row, have let someone step in front of you in a queue, have taken on a colleague's work to keep in with him, have accepted a repair bill you were afraid to challenge, have not dared to ask out a girl or boy who attracts you.

Having made your list, tackle each item individually, taking the easiest first. If, for instance, you are anxiously trying to please everyone at work, try, once, to refuse to take on extra work for a colleague. Once you have established a precedent, it will make it easier the next time. Assertiveness training does not mean walking into your boss's office and having a stand-up row about a salary rise: it is a conscious, gentle change of behaviour, aimed at reducing your anxiety about coping.

CONTROLLING OBSESSIVE FEARS

Once obsessive-compulsive rituals have become a way of life, psychiatric help is needed to overcome them. But their onset is usually noticed – by a partner, colleague or flatmate. One woman, who spent hours a day compulsively rewashing clothes and bedwear, told me she was quite unaware of her growing preoccupation with cleanliness until her husband asked her in a puzzled way why she was washing up the cups twice. At a very early stage, you can aim at changing your own behaviour. If you have been spending time checking your clothes, washing your hands constantly to avoid contamination, or rigidly carrying out any other acts – and are genuinely fearful as to what will happen if you do not – then try to change your behaviour. Leave clothes deliberately untidy, kitchen appliances unchecked, a few dishes unwashed. It may well bring on an anxiety attack, but this is containable. The alternative is a life increasingly preoccupied with ritual hand-washing or checking.

RECOVERY

Anxiety and stress are the products of your living or working conditions and your relationships, or lack of them. Tranquillisers may help you over a particular crisis; learning to relax, and other techniques, can help reduce the physical sensations anxiety creates. But these may just act as a 'holding operation'. The fundamental reason behind the stress needs to be found, acknowledged and tackled if the anxiety and fears are to end.

5

Depression

'My depression started when I was twenty. I'd had a boyfriend for six years and then met another man I liked. I was confused about which to marry. It got in the end I just wanted to get out of it all and I attempted suicide as a way out. Then, when I did marry, I lived in a house that was rotting away and again I got very depressed.

'When I get depressed I feel that even on the sunniest day the world looks black. I wish I could just escape into an obscurity and look forward to eternal blackness. By nature I'm an extrovert and very bubbly and I hide depression by talking a lot and laughing. I can be with people who don't know anything about it, but on my own it's sometimes so bad I just wish I was dead.

'I have two children, I work for half the day. I go out with friends regularly, my house is nice. I love my husband very much. My mother died three years ago and afterwards I got very depressed, for I adored her. Since then I have been more depressed than ever. I'm afraid I sometimes drink a lot, but it doesn't help.

'I don't want to get up at all. Nothing I do makes me happy. The slightest thing sends me into a rage. I feel I try very hard to combat it. I've taken on all sorts of varied hobbies, but once finished I feel very depressed.

'On occasions when I can't sleep and feel very disturbed, I've rung the Samaritans. Only I feel that's not long-standing help on the days when life seems so useless to me. My husband is very good but must get fed up with coming home to find me in tears. When I get depressed I drive my own car. I want to drive away for ever, where to God knows. The worst of depression is that you don't want people. I don't answer the phone if I'm really bad, and I shake in the hands. I also bite my fingers till they bleed, but I just can't stop.'

Many of those suffering from depression have experienced feelings like those of the woman quoted above. Like her, their attitude is negative. This is understandable. Depression attacks the will – the will to look on the positive side or to take any positive action to change your outlook or circumstances. It is a painful and debilitating experience, when you get mentally locked into yourself, examining every possible cause for your depression, and feeling increasingly inadequate. With this negative and self-critical attitude of mind, no realistic evaluation is ever made. Fatigue, lethargy and lack of confidence make decisions impossible. The exasperation of partners, relations or friends worsens matters by creating guilt.

A great many people are helped by psychotherapy, drugs or electroconvulsive therapy (ECT), but some people who suffer from depression also find it helpful to share their experiences with fellow sufferers and in this way reduce their sense of isolation. Quite often, drug treatment may be usefully combined with psychotherapy. And, equally, a person being treated medically or by therapy may also find the support of a self-help group invaluable. Consistent support and encouragement from within the group helps others to recover.

Self-help and mutual help groups run on these lines – working alongside conventional medicine, and offering a supporting service to those who have recovered but still need help, or did not benefit from the treatment – can be very valuable. (*More information about groups set up in the belief that depressives can help themselves by helping each other is in the section Self-help groups.*)

Much of this chapter is about other people's experiences of depression. This is because so many feel isolated within their depression and believe that no one else can understand or share their emotions. Identifying with others who have had the same experiences and causes behind their depression helps them feel less cut off; reveals how widespread such feelings are; and helps others, unaffected by depression, to understand a little of what it can be like. At certain stages of depression, however, reading about others similarly situated has an adverse effect. Those who feel this way should turn to the reassuring, practical sections at the end of this chapter.

Depression is a word that has too many shades of meaning. It's used lightly to describe 'the blues' and, at the other end of the spectrum, to describe a black, hopeless despair which can lead to suicide: a state when, as one psychiatrist put it, 'the self seems worthless, the outer world meaningless and the future hopeless'.

Traditionally, most psychiatrists consider that there are two types of depression: *reactive* and *endogenous*. A reactive depression is one that is triggered by a traumatic life event. An endogenous depression is one that arises spontaneously, with no apparent external cause. In reality, these distinctions are probably not quite so clear-cut, in that most depressive illnesses probably arise out of a combination of both factors. That is to say that a person who is constitutionally prone to depression may develop the illness as a result of a life event which a more robust person will manage to cope with. Stuart Sutherland, in his partly autobiographical book *Breakdown*, says that he was told by his psychiatrist: 'It does not matter whether we call your illness reactive depression or endogenous depression, the treatment is the same.'

Psychiatrists stress that it is important to distinguish between unhappiness and depression. ('People seem to expect drugs to cure their broken marriages,' said one.) There are many who have unhappy experiences and there are others who have difficulties in coping with their life or their work. These find it hard to form or maintain relationships. They are depressed at their inadequacy to manage, and aware that the cause is their own personality deficiencies. Their 'depression' needs to be helped by emotional and practical support: they need to build up a network of friends to help them through bad patches, when they feel too inadequate to cope; they need to avoid overstretching themselves at work and bringing on nervous strain. Some form of counselling or psychotherapy can help reveal why someone, for example, constantly gets involved with married partners or aggression at work. Personal inadequacies cannot be solved by antidepressants: a different kind of help is needed.

However, if a cluster of emotionally upsetting events occurs, those who are not so tough may develop a depressive illness. This may be because of a severe grief reaction in the case of a bereavement, for example; or it may trigger off a chemically based predisposition to depression. Whatever the label put on the depression, treatment is now needed.

Of the five hundred or so sufferers I spoke to, or whose letters I read, many knew why they were depressed, though could not fight it; others were less able to explain their feelings of despair. Their experiences show how universal depression is, and reveal some of the symptoms of this illness, examples of its onset and causes, and the effects of treatment.

SYMPTOMS

Depression is a way of mentally withdrawing oneself from a situation or surroundings that are impossible to accept, or cope with, any longer. It usually produces a mixture of the following disorders: loss of appetite – or occasionally excess eating; headaches; constipation; lack of concentration or muzziness; insomnia; poor memory; sense of guilt or self-blame; feelings of unworthiness; fears of ill-health, ranging from mild illness to, say, cancer, loss of sexual interest; difficulty in thinking; sadness with low self-esteem; suicidal ideas and behaviour; self-absorption, with reduced interest in surroundings; heightening of personality traits – that is, a person might get *more* anxious, obsessional, phobic, hypochondriacal or paranoid.

One wife, describing her husband's symptoms, said: 'He wakes up every morning, deeply depressed; lies in bed most of the day; on arising, sleeps in his chair, even if anyone should call; does not wish to speak to people; makes for the nearest chair when shopping and falls asleep; is deeply depressed every day; is not interested in anything or his appearance; has no conversation and all decisions have to be made by me. He has a fluttering on his chest and his stomach churns over every day; he has lost a lot of weight.'

Similar feelings of inertia were expressed by others. 'I am so very sick of this half-dead feeling and almost complete inability to enjoy anything,' said one middle-aged woman. 'I feel so cut off from everyone. The everlasting effect of trying to appear bright and cheerful is such a strain. I try to hide it from the family.' Another housewife said:

'A sense of isolation is gradually taking over my life. I find myself unable, and sometimes unwilling, to approach other people.'

It is particularly sad when such feelings affect young people, leaving them without even the memory of stability and happiness. One girl of nineteen said the severe depression she suffered from had built up over the years since she was sixteen: 'It brings terrible feelings of isolation, loneliness and bouts of despair. It makes me feel like a social outcast.' This was echoed by a young girl of fifteen, who said, 'I never attempt to go out, but sit around the house all day except when I go to school, and I can't go there often. I have been tempted to attempt suicide many times.'

One young man, who had had long bouts of mild depression when he was a teenager, had gone on to university and found that his depression worsened: 'I was having very bad sleeping difficulties and it was coming up to the time that I had to make a decision about what to do the following year and I couldn't get myself interested in doing anything. I also felt increasingly cut off. I often went to parties and felt "not there".' He was often defeated by the mere effort of getting up in the morning: 'You stay in bed for days, not exactly afraid to get up, but unable to summon the energy to get around to it. All the normal tasks take for ever: you are defeated by the idea of frying an egg. It would be nice if someone realised what an achievement it is to get up and get washed: it sounds ridiculous, but one of the most extraordinary things about depression is this fantastic lassitude.'

These general feelings of lassitude, so prevalent in depression, often disguise what is happening. People looking after ageing parents, or young children, expect to feel tired, and are unaware that it could herald the gradual onset of depression. One woman in her early twenties, with two young children, said it had taken a year before she realised that there was anything wrong. 'You feel very disillusioned with life and the world and your family, and not much use to anyone. Things seem to get blacker and blacker. When I got up in the morning, I really faced a very pleasant day ahead; yet I dreaded getting up. All my confidence went, I hated being in the house on my own for the fear of what I might do, and the silence drove me mad. I was far happier in other people's houses and company. I used to work one day a week and would dread going home; but I couldn't understand that as everything I cared for and loved was at home. I think it was having to face up to my responsibility.

'I remember dreading my son's birthday. When the children all arrived, I had this terrible shaking feeling that I couldn't cope. I asked my husband to be there and I remember bursting into tears and him coming in and saying, "Pull yourself together" and being very cross.

'I did not know what to do with my time and, if a day lay ahead of me, it seemed such a long day. How was I to cope? I felt as if I had to have something to do all the time, to keep my mind from wandering off into suicide. I never tried to commit suicide, but contemplated it. What stopped me was the children finding me: my strength was their need of me. But I did not want to live: everything was very passive and dead. I felt if I did not wake up, I wouldn't have to face another day – what a relief! I had a terrible fear of being alone and did not want to bother to put on make-up or dress, or buy any new clothes.

'One particular Sunday I remember that we went for a walk and on our return I just cried and cried and cried. At that time – about eighteen months after these feelings had first begun – I suppose I had reached a crisis. I probably needed a doctor, but I wasn't keen. Then in desperation I went to see the family planning doctor, because I wanted to know if it was the pill. I cried all the time I was seeing the clinic doctor. It was so embarrassing. She suggested I came off the pill and I did, but it did not help. I went to my own doctor finally and he said, "Are you having husband trouble?" And I thought, he hasn't got the time to talk to me.

'I got up daily, not wanting to live, not thinking I was important to the children. All I knew was if I stayed in the house and not keep going, I would do something dreadful. You try to think positively, but you worry about all those things in your mind, and yet you don't know what you're worrying about.

'I clung to my husband an awful lot, but he couldn't stand it. It made him reject me and made me feel ten times worse. He turned a blind eye and hoped it would all go away and this frightened me very much. If we had a late night, I kept going for my husband's sake. It is probably why he did not take it seriously. I used to shake and dread a late night. I always felt ten times worse through lack of sleep, and went to pieces the next day.

'I can remember thinking, "Why are people so happy?" Because there was nothing to be cheerful about. I was very passive. I'm normally enthusiastic, and when I am angry I shout; but at that time I just stayed on the same level. I'd get into a panic about the simplest things, like coping with the washing and ironing. But I kept making myself do it and, however bad I felt, I got up to do the basic things. I just forced myself. The people who did not know me did not know that anything was really wrong.

'Although I did not think I was very strong, I must have been to have kept on going like that. I might have an hour or two in the day when I felt all right and then I would go back into it. But gradually and slowly I began to feel better. I was as slow getting out of it as I was getting into it. One of the things that helped me was hearing my six-year-old son say to my husband, "Aren't we lucky, Daddy, Mummy hasn't been crying so much lately." I knew my crying must upset the children, and I really tried not to. There was this cold deadness about everything, but this remark broke through. I thought, I must get well just to help them through their school life: perhaps they do need me after all. I also managed to help someone else who was depressed. She kept ringing me up and it was a relief to come across someone else.'

These feelings of inadequacy and inability to cope were one of the most often mentioned symptoms of depression. One man of forty-one with three children, who had suffered from depression since fifteen, said, 'I can't seem to raise my head out of my hands to fight back against life. My confidence has gone, I don't work. Sometimes I catch a bus and go for a long ride out into the country.'

Another girl admitted to having given up her job, though knowing this was unwise, because she could not cope any longer. 'Even the small degree of responsibility that this involved was too much for me. I was terrified someone would ask me to do something and I would just crumple into tears. I was losing weight, and having constant headaches and indigestion. I know that to mix keeps me in touch with life, but it is not easy.'

The withdrawal from society can be very pronounced. 'My son married three years ago,' said one mother, 'and is under treatment for severe depression. He doesn't work, can't mix at all with people. If anybody calls, it's so difficult to converse, as he barely opens his mouth.'

This isolation can easily lead to morbid fears and doubts. 'My father now mistrusts those close to him,' said another woman, 'and keeps asking when the doctors are coming to take him away. He stays in the bedroom as much as possible, away from other people. He's lost interest in everything.'

The family in this case were understandably feeling the strain, and were trying to break down the father's isolation by getting people to visit him. To stay alone in one's room is not accepted as 'normal' social behaviour: there is immediate pressure put on the person concerned to mix, to conform to the social habits of everyone else. This attitude, to the person concerned, only underlines his conviction that other people have no understanding of how he feels.

As one woman in her early forties said: 'No one who has not suffered from depression can believe what it is like. It is as if someone or something takes you over and you just don't seem to have control over what you do or how you feel. When you have depression, you really do think you are the only one who has felt that miserable or that guilty. It is like going through a long tunnel and you just cannot find the way out, or the other side. Instead of thinking things can't get worse, you think you are to blame for the way you feel and nobody else can help. You certainly are not capable of helping yourself, so things can only go from bad to worse.'

Depression is sometimes accepted as a 'punishment' for something that may have happened in the past, so often brings with it feelings of guilt. As one woman said: 'I accept my depression now and feel one has to learn to live with it, with an overwhelming sense of guilt about the past, self-hatred. I have to adjust to the fact that I cannot put things right, cannot relive the past and do things differently.' Another agreed: 'I do not seem to be able to overcome these guilt feelings; this self-punishment thing is getting me down. Nobody knows how I mutilate myself. I'm getting very frightened as these suicidal tendencies I've got are getting very strong.'

Another common occurrence in depression is the conviction that the signs of stress affecting one's body – such as palpitations – are serious physical symptoms of illness. This, in turn, increases the depression. One woman's depression worsened after she became convinced she was going to die of heart trouble. Her eldest daughter took her to hospital, and begged them to do something. They gave her a thorough examination, but found nothing wrong physically, and told her her illness was all in the mind. 'She isn't convinced,' said the daughter. 'She doesn't take much interest in the family and seems only interested in herself. She also has some varicose veins and thread veins in her face and these, to her, are more reasons why she should hide herself away.'

CAUSES

Depression is generally accepted as being caused by changes in body chemistry and/or by 'life events'. Inheritance may play a part, and so may childhood, by creating an anxious, vulnerable personality.

BODY CHEMISTRY

Research has shown that the level of certain substances in the brain falls during depression (a reason why antidepressants, by raising these levels, counteract depression). However, it is not proved that the lowered level of these substances *causes* the depression: it may equally be caused *by* the depression. There are also other theories of chemical predisposition. For example, Merton Sandler, Professor of Chemical Pathology at London University, has been testing whether people with a vulnerability to depression show abnormalities in the way they break down a substance called tyramine, present in ordinary foods. Whether or not the person is depressed at the time, the abnormality will be there – predisposing them to depression.

EVENTS

Events in themselves can cause depression. They can also trigger off depression in those predisposed towards it, either chemically or through personality.

It is of practical importance, therefore, to look at the type of event that can cause the onset of depression.

George W. Brown and Tirril Harris, in their detailed research into a group of depressed women in south London, reported in their book *Social Origins of Depression*, found that it was not just any event, however upsetting, that could bring about depression. Only certain severe events, involving a long-term threat, could do so. For instance, even the emotional trauma of a child nearly dying was not as significant in causing the onset of depression as a prolonged condition such as overcrowded, damp housing.

The distinctive feature of most of such long-term events, they found, 'is the experience of loss or disappointment, if this is defined broadly to include threat of or actual separation from a key figure; an unpleasant revelation about someone close, a life-threatening illness to a close relative, a major material loss or general disappointment or threat of them, and miscellaneous crises such as being made redundant after a long period of steady employment'. Quite minor events could also cause depression if they brought home the hopelessness of a person's position. One woman, for example, who was living in bad housing, became depressed after her sister's engagement.

Brown and Harris also found that depression was linked to social class: working-class women with children at home were four times more likely to develop depression when a severe event or major difficulty occurred. This was not just due to being subject to more stress, like money problems, but to what they call 'vulnerability factors'. These factors do not themselves cause depression, but make a woman more vulnerable to depression.

The first factor which puts a woman at risk is the lack of someone, such as an understanding husband or boyfriend, in whom she can trust and confide. The second is having three or more children aged under fourteen living at home. The third is the loss of a mother (though not father) before reaching eleven years. The fourth is lack of employment outside the home (which, apart from the interest of a job, broadens the chance of making other social contacts). If these vulnerability factors apply, and a severe life event then takes place, the likelihood of depression is almost 100 per cent.

BEREAVEMENT AND LOSS

In talking to people with depression, the 'experience of loss' – which Brown and Harris use in a broad context, covering separation, divorce and loss of job, as well as bereavement – is particularly evident.

A woman in her late forties said that she had lost her husband nearly three years ago, and still could not believe it or accept it. 'I used to be the life and soul of everything: now I don't want to eat, shop or anything. I am irritable and can't make a decision. I have seen doctors and specialists, but nothing helps me.' Other bereaved people have also stopped in this time vacuum: 'I've felt dead inside ever since'; 'I seem to have lost all interest in life and always feel tired'; 'My mother sits and cries for hours since the death of my father two years ago: she neglects the home and herself and feels alone and terrified. The only thing that stops her from committing suicide is her conviction that she will not see my father again if she does.' Another woman, after her husband had died comparatively young in his fifties, said that life, for her, had stopped. 'Where I live there are no neighbours, not even a light at night. I am a mile from the bus stop. Life just isn't worth living any more.'

Bereavement can bring on feelings of guilt and lack of self-regard, as well as sorrow. One mother, for instance, had a breakdown after her husband died of cancer, and went into psychiatric hospital for electrical shock treatment. Her three small children were then taken into care. Now a day patient, she is still very depressed, most of all at night. 'The doctors tell me to go out at night and make friends. But as a woman I can't go out on my own; I would feel cheap. They don't understand. Every night there's the same empty house, cigarettes and the television. I took an overdose recently and I feel that I can't go on much longer. I see the children at the weekend, but they won't let me keep them overnight. But I can't blame them. I'm not fit to be a mother.'

For help with bereavement, contact your local social services department and see if there is any form of bereavement counselling available. If not, ask your doctor if he can recommend a counsellor or psychotherapist who works in your area and can see you. After a bereavement there is a very great need to talk out your feelings, and to recall memories. Sometimes a person may feel guilt, which needs to be discussed rather than repressed. There is bound to be loneliness. Too often, after the funeral is over, friends and neighbours tend to avoid the bereaved person out of embarrassment or anxiety over what to say. Yet it is a time when as much companionship as possible is needed, and should be offered. Mutual-help organisations can also be of great help here (see Appendix II).

'LOSS' OF CHILDREN

Naturally, widows and widowers who have brought up children feel doubly lonely and depressed when they, in turn, leave. 'My daughter left this town to live in Wales,' said one woman, 'and I do so miss her and the children's company. Then I had to have my dog put to sleep. I am losing interest in the home and I have no energy.'

Even those who are still married can feel an almost equal sense of loss. 'I am a redundant mother,' said another woman. 'I have been living my life through my children, helping them to shape their careers. When they left home to go to college, I could not identify myself with anyone. I have felt for years that I do not know who I am or what I want out of life. My husband being indifferent to all this and not understanding made me feel more guilty and unworthy than ever. Then my son, with whom I had a warm and humorous relationship, married and his wife said it was wrong for a mother and son to have such a bond between them and she would do what she could to break it up. My son has changed so much that I cannot believe it. I feel it is my fault. All the men in my life reject me.'

Unlike a bereavement, it is at least known in advance that children will leave home. This still does not help with the loneliness when it happens, but deliberately getting involved with other activities a few years in advance prevents too much time being spent on brooding about the loss of the children.

DIVORCE AND SEPARATION

These feelings of rejection are naturally particularly strong among those who have been divorced or separated. 'At twenty-eight,' said one woman, 'I feel there should be something good in life somewhere. There used to be until my husband ran off and left us. Now I feel there is nothing and the trouble is I feel it will always be like this. I cannot visualise anything else, ever. The future seems like an endless black pit and the past like hell.'

A woman of sixty, whose husband had left her after forty years of marriage, said: 'I had a busy life, working as a secretary and bringing up a child, until we retired here two years ago. I miss my marriage, I miss my work and I find it very difficult to reorganise my lonely life. I am going through a period of depression and need help.' One divorced woman was worried about the effect her depression was having on her children: 'My daughter of twenty-one hardly goes out and doesn't mix with people. My teenage son is a loner. The children cannot forgive their father: they go quite distant and shut themselves up. How long must this go on for us all?' Teenagers are particularly vulnerable to emotional shock. One girl of seventeen, whose boyfriend married another girl, became withdrawn and tearful, refusing to go out of the house to local clubs, because she felt a failure.

Men are equally susceptible to feelings of rejection. One middle-aged man, whose wife had left him and his two young children, said that he had tried to fight back the depression this had caused him, but feeling lonely and rejected he had attempted to form another relationship. He met a girl, who was also separated, but decided that her children and his would, together, be too much to cope with. Long hours at his job, a financial necessity, added to his stress. 'I completely went to pieces, became severely depressed, and now go to the doctor's constantly. I do less hours at work, and seem to have lost interest in everything. I weep a lot and at times feel I wish I could end it all, but the children keep me going.'

Many who are separated or divorced make the same point about their children. One woman said: 'I know rejection, ECT, absolute despair, the run-away feeling, the lonely days, not speaking to a soul from morning till evening. I've kept myself asleep with drugs for days on end. I've had as many as two hundred sleeping pills here at home at one time. Why I didn't take them all at once was that my lovely young daughter was constantly in my mind. But how can I stop feeling so hopeless? There's no confidence in me now. I never go into the town even to do the shopping. I drive to the nearest village, so that no one I know can see me as I am now. Conversation is out of the question. I spend nearly all day in bed: food is not important to me.'

'Each new day is like the day before,' said one widow. 'You shop alone, eat alone, sit alone in despair until it is time to turn to your only friend, the sleeping pill. We are given plenty of good advice, like join some club. But we don't all have a club near, and we can't all face up to walking into a club alone.'

For those who cannot face joining a mixed club, or going into a pub alone, church activities or a single-sex club such as bowls or cookery might provide an alternative. Classes such as pottery or painting are also less obviously social. Although 'joining a club' has become a cliché, it is still a good way of passing the time and alleviating loneliness.

UNEMPLOYMENT, REDUNDANCY

Losing one's job, a long period of redundancy, or early retirement can bring on equal feelings of hopelessness. 'My husband was a man at the top of his field in his salesman career,' said one woman. 'But, after a nervous breakdown and a try at working again after three months, he had eventually to admit defeat and retire early. Since that time, he has deteriorated rapidly into deep depression because he feels a worthless, useless member of society.'

The sense of inadequacy and depression brought on by failing to get work can be very strong. 'I couldn't possibly feel any worse than I do,' said one young teacher, who had applied unsuccessfully for over forty teaching posts. A man of nearly sixty, in another instance, lost the job at which he had worked for nearly forty years. He got another job fairly quickly, but it was work of which he had no previous experience. After a time, this lack of experience began to give him a feeling of incompetence, particularly as he was working with younger people. He would start to shake in the presence of other people at work, increasingly lacked concentration and had feelings of panic. He was finally sacked and had to register as unemployed. His symptoms intensified, he could hardly face any interviews, and he was overcome by feelings of hopelessness.

The erosion of self-confidence in being without a job, and aware of being at home all day when others are working, can be very serious, affecting other areas of life, such as personal relationships. Waiting for the 'right' job can entail being at home for months, even years, while the will or ability to work gets whittled away. Any job, even one of just an hour or so a day, is a way of keeping in contact with people. A doctor or Citizens' Advice Bureau should be able to suggest a counsellor or psychotherapist if you feel unable to cope unaided.

PRESSURE AT WORK

Pressures at work can also induce stress which, in turn, brings on depression. One man, who had worked in a store for seven years without a day's illness, was hard-working, but sensitive to criticism. Because of problems at work he suddenly had a breakdown. He changed his job and was initially very keen at his new job – but after a week at home, due to a minor traffic accident, he could not face returning to work. He changed his job again, but now finds that an almost unmanageable depression sets in after any break from routine, especially after holidays and on Monday mornings.

In another case, a young girl, who changed her job to one where she had to work 'with one of the most awful women you could imagine,' developed sickness and pains in her chest. She also got very tired and tense, started crying a lot and lost weight. Although she ultimately changed her job, even the ensuing part-time one she took on made her so tired that it brought back the depression.

Too much pressure at work can cause panic attacks and stress-related illnesses. You usually know if you are carrying too much responsibility or if relationships with colleagues are moving to a crisis point. If you are unable to delegate work, or to face a likely confrontation, it is better to change your job before illness – mental or stress-related – forces you to do so.

PREDISPOSITION

Many express total bewilderment at a depression which, to them, is incomprehensible. 'I can't say I have any real worries,' said one woman. 'The family are grown up, we have a comfortable home, even if not a luxurious one; we aren't really on the breadline. But this feeling of despair descends on me. I just feel as though there isn't a purpose in life.'

Another woman said: 'I am in my thirties, have two gorgeous children and am of reasonable appearance. I have nothing really to complain about apart from separating from my husband, whom I still care about very much. But I know a lot of the main cause for our parting rested with my outlook on life. No matter how I reason with myself, depression always seems to get the best of me and everything just becomes a thorough waste of time. I become a repulsive nothing, and the home a prison. Everything suffers regularly and life becomes one exhausting fight. The heartbreaking thing is that I know what I am doing, but, God, where do you get the power to stop it?'

For many, depression comes in cycles. 'For me, it is always July and August,' said one man. 'I can feel it coming on. The world feels dead, and so do I. It has happened this way for years.' Winston Churchill suffered from this type of depression, calling it 'my black dog'.

Those with recurring or cyclical depression need to go for treatment as soon as they are conscious of the signs of its appearance. They need to talk to the doctor or psychiatrist about how long and how often these episodes are likely to be. If they are reasonably mild, contact with a self-help and mutual help support group could be very helpful at these times.

MANIC DEPRESSION

A minority of people suffer from manic depression – that is, extreme cycles from agitated, euphoric behaviour (mania) to periods of deep depression. Many more of us have rather milder swings of mood.

One young girl who had suffered from mood swings for several years said: 'I swing from high elation which lasts five or six months, then go down and become withdrawn and depressed. I have very few friends, as this has a great effect on relationships. When I'm up, I'm full of fun, efficient at work, tidy and organised. When I'm down, I'm very quiet, no sense of humour, untidy, confused and slow. It is difficult to explain to others why you cannot cope with your job so well: people cannot understand why I cannot laugh and chatter. My parents, who try hard to support me, and who will do anything to see me well, are beginning to feel the strain and tension.'

In the euphoric stage, sufferers can experience feelings of marked cheerfulness, wild hilarity, and excitement, and may also carry out unpredictable actions. They are likely to be overactive and restless. They have a rapid stream of thought; they talk constantly; their attention is intense, but fleeting; they are distracted by trivial events, and start projects without completing them. They also think they have the world at their feet, getting through vast sums of money, whether they possess any or not. (One psychiatric nurse received a telephone call from an airline, verifying whether Mr X, one of his hypomanic patients, was in a position to buy a Boeing 707.)

'As far as friends, relations or a partner are concerned,' said one psychiatrist, 'the manic phase is more likely than the depressive phase to cause them panic and anxiety as it's pretty overpowering. The person is likely to sit up all day and run around all night; and they can do damaging things to themselves socially and financially. They might pack in their job, and spend all their money in about half a day, ending up with £100,000 of debts on credit. They may become aggressive. People who are manic cannot be thwarted and under those circumstances they will knock you down. But they are so distractable that you can change the subject very easily.'

The strain of living with a partner or relative in these circumstances can be intense. One woman spoke of a friend of hers whose husband had suffered this way for some fifteen years: 'She appears on my doorstep, tense, strung up, often in tears and so distressed she can hardly stand up. She has sleeping pills and tranquillisers to help her over the bad patches, but these are occurring more often and she resents having to resort to drugs just to live in the same house as her husband. Sometimes he carries out his threats to do odd things, such as selling some of the furniture and pulling all the kitchen fitments off the wall. He even threatened to sell the home.'

Many sufferers stress the awareness they have of going in and out of their cycles of mood. 'It's like plunging through a quicksand,' said one young man of twenty-six. 'You notice it more coming out of depression than going into it: the way black clouds move away and you get the feeling that the sun is coming out from behind them. Suddenly you are in the same world as everyone else, and everything has a different slant. You appreciate such simple things: you get a tremendous kick out of commuting in on the train. It sounds grotesque, but it's really amazing. It's a very physical feeling. I remember my wife once had to take my cheque book, because when I went manic I would buy the most ridiculous things. I would stay on the crest of a wave, and then suddenly plunge down the other side.'

Another twenty-year-old girl, who had suffered bouts of depression every ten months or so since she was fourteen, said: 'They usually have a three-week build-up, when I become what I term "an emotional see-saw", going up and down from minute to minute. One moment I can be deliriously happy and within ten minutes I want to cry. I then have two to three weeks of deep depression when I cry almost constantly and have to take time off work because I am incapable. Everything seems too much trouble. Slowly the depression lifts, taking two to three weeks before I feel able to relax on my own.'

Similar feelings were expressed by a middle-aged man: 'I normally can't mix or get on with people, unless I'm on one of my "high" periods, when I can meet the world and talk non-stop to anyone and everyone. But though I still occasionally get these very brief periods of unbounded optimism and euphoria, when I'm capable of anything and life is sheer ecstasy, ninety-five per cent of the time now, it's utter depression.'

CYCLES

The cycles of elation and depression vary individually in both how long they last and how often they recur. The likelihood of recovery from an individual attack is good. As a patient grows older, the depressive attacks become more common than manic ones.

TREATMENT

One of the most widely used treatments is lithium carbonate, as it reduces the severity of both the depression and the mania. Lithium can be found naturally in many mineral springs (it was advocated as a cure for gout in the last century). In the 1940s, experiments showed its stabilising nature on patients suffering from mania and in recent years research has indicated that it also reduces the level of depression. As there is a narrow margin between good and bad effects when it is administered, the amount of lithium in the body has to be measured carefully through blood samples – several checks weekly being required initially. Because the treatment is long-term, lithium is not prescribed unless it is thought essential to deal with recurrent attacks. Major tranquillisers are usually tried first.

Research is being carried out – mainly in America – on multivitamin therapy in connection with severe mood swings; and Dr Richard Mackarness, author of *Not All in the Mind*, has also found that food allergies can play an important part. One woman who said that she was 'having mood swings from elation to severe depression, and burning myself with cigarettes' was admitted to hospital and given psychotherapy, which was unsuccessful. The registrar gave her up as hopeless after five weeks and referred her to Dr Richard Mackarness. He put her on a strict diet for a week – fresh meat and vegetables only, and just water to drink. She was tested, and found to be allergic to white flour, sugar, tea, instant coffee and egg white. 'The result was that I was discharged with no drugs, except one as standby which I rarely need. As long as I stick to my diet, I'm fine.'

SUGGESTIONS

1   Those with severe mood swings are frequently very reluctant to seek help, since they find that life is very grey without the elated periods, and they do not consider themselves ill. Advice may have to

be sought from the doctor with regard to treatment. It may be that a counsellor can help in showing the person that his behaviour is causing the destruction of family life and possibly the break-up of the marriage, and that treatment is essential.

2 Ways of testing for allergies are contained in Dr Mackarness's book, but these must be undertaken only with the co-operation of the family doctor.

3 Children are understandably confused by the apparently different personalities of the parent, particularly if the parents are overprotective and never talk about it. An open discussion is far healthier if the children are old enough to understand. Counselling or therapy work with the family is often necessary, if it is to come through. A local Family Service Unit or family therapy can help here; so can a social worker or a community psychiatric nurse.

4 If the side-effects of lithium or constant maintenance on this drug are unacceptable to the patient, one answer has been for patients to enter into agreements (virtually 'contracts') with their medical practitioner that they will guarantee to recommence lithium treatment at the first sign of the recurrence of their illness.

5 The meetings run by some of the local associations of MIND may present an opportunity of meeting others who are caring for or living with sufferers, and of discussing mutual problems.

ADOLESCENT DEPRESSION

Adolescence is usually characterised by intense and often volatile emotions. Thus a teenager may experience depression much more intensely than an older person. One teenager said that, in taking A levels, she had been under a great deal of pressure to succeed, and this had been coupled with an unhappy family background. Her depression had been triggered off by something a friend had said to her. 'Within one month, from being quite an active person, I became totally disabled, not being able to perform the most menial of tasks. I couldn't think or understand the simplest things people were saying, I could only think of suicide.'

A mother of another young girl, who had been acutely depressed for six months and was in and out of hospital, was completely bemused by the situation. 'She has a good job, is financially secure, has good friends and, really, on the face of it, nothing to worry about. We are really at a loss to know what to do next and the suspense is getting us down, as both my husband and I are elderly.' Parents are often taken unaware by their children's feelings. One father said: 'Our son of eighteen is suffering from depression. It showed itself a few months ago when he went out in the snow and swallowed a lot of tablets plus various drinks. This was the first indication we had that anything was wrong. The trouble continued on and off until he walked out of the house and slept rough for two nights. He has failed his exams and now just hangs around the house.'

Adolescents may find it hard to talk to their doctor, or parents; many find it easier to share their problems with their contemporaries, with whom they can identify, and who are removed from the family circle.

One Samaritan helper at that organisation's London headquarters, said that in 1978 they had over 500 calls from adolescents of sixteen and under. He stressed that it is often not realised that young people of that age can get just as depressed as older ones. He thinks that many of the fourteen- and fifteen-year-olds who get in touch with them do so because of a background of relationship problems with parents who are divorced or separated; emotional problems with boyfriends or girlfriends, especially teenage pregnancies; difficulties at school in connection with exams; or bullying. Asian teenagers often have problems over the restrictions put on them by their parents. One reason why more young people are going to the Samaritans may be that it is more acceptable to ask for help nowadays, to be more open about relationship problems, instead of just keeping a stiff upper lip. 'But there is a kind of despair which is around,' said the Samaritan. 'A person's spirits go up and down. The tolerance of stress varies and some personalities are vulnerable.'

LONELINESS

Young people, particularly those from broken homes, can find it difficult to make personal relationships and friendships. This in itself creates depression which is, in turn, worsened by loneliness. Yet the loneliness sometimes felt within marriage can be as bad, if not worse, than that experienced by someone living alone. 'We have just moved to the country', said one woman, 'and I do not know a soul. I never exchange a word with anyone. I've tried to get a job, but with a little boy at school it's impossible. I've got problems with my marriage which I could not have foreseen and I am really at the end of my tether with loneliness.' Another woman said: 'I feel lonely, although I have three children, and a husband. I hate being alone, and also I get very easily upset by my husband. I am beginning to feel just awful and I have so little confidence.'

In another case, a woman had been receiving psychiatric treatment for five years, without improving, because the situation which was causing it remained the same. 'My husband works permanent nights. I cannot go out very often leaving two children under school age, so really I stay at home all the time, maybe having a night out once every two or three weeks. I have no friends in the area where I live.'

Sometimes the aura of depression surrounding a person makes other people back away, almost as if it were a physical disease which they could catch. 'I seem to have no friends and my family stay away,' said one woman who was being treated for depression. 'I've found it difficult to put over to them how I feel.'

Those with established depression cannot be told to 'make friends with the neighbours', as once depression has taken hold they feel too worthless and inadequate to make friends. For these reasons, people's attempts to make friends with them are likely to be repulsed. Anti-depressants can sometimes help lift the mood long enough to provide enough impetus to make contact with neighbours. A woman's group or asking the Samaritans for a 'befriender' can help here.

ENVIRONMENT

The isolation and stress caused by tower-block living and other bad housing conditions is a well-known cause of depression. This is, understandably, because those concerned can see no way out of it.

'I asked the council to move me as this flat is up so many steps,' said one man. 'I can't see out of the windows, it's so high it's like living in a jail. It's a very depressing place.' Moving to a tower block for another girl cemented the depression that had begun when she ended her engagement because her fiancé was dating another woman. Shortly after the move, her father had a heart attack and hurt his back in a fall, so was in a wheelchair. 'We don't have any friends, you don't seem to make them. The old pair who live above know my father is like he is and they give us a hell of a life, banging down on the floor all day. When I went up to ask if they could give us some peace, she slammed the door in my face and then sent her husband down when he had a few drinks. What does one do when you're so down and can't get up or see any way out? Life seems so pointless.'

Another woman had similar problems where she lived: 'One reason why I am so depressed is because I cannot make friends easily. I am too afraid to talk to people and when I try I just don't know what to say. I live a long way from my childhood home and from my one lifelong friend. I am unhappy where I live for other reasons. My home is in the middle of a long row of terrace houses which are very old. Residents have a communal right of way past everybody else's doorstep. The backs of the houses are a disgrace: unkempt patches of mud and broken-down fences. It looks a slum. The walls of the houses inside are very thin and you can hear what's going on in the early hours of the morning. One side, they are only a young couple with one child and every other night he comes home drunk and beats her up: the screaming is terrible. I am nearly driven out of my mind because I cannot let my two small children out to play without constant vigilance. I have begged my husband to make our little patch into a lawn, but he doesn't seem to feel there is any urgency in this matter.

'I lived till marriage out in the country and cannot get used to living in an industrial city. Everything gets coal black, even the soil in the garden, and I feel deeply upset that my beautiful children should have to be brought up in this area. I am beginning to cry again very easily and my children then get distressed.'

Vandalised estates, vendettas with neighbours, women screaming because of husbands or boyfriends beating them up, walls 'like tissue paper', lack of friends – all are high on the list of reasons people give to account for their depression. And recognising the problems doesn't help if apparently nothing can be done. 'I had severe depression three years ago,' said one young wife, 'I was cooped up in a tiny flat with two toddlers, with my husband away a lot working, and my mother-in-law to look after. I stayed in hospital for about eight weeks and came right back to the same "environmental" problems. These have increased with another baby, inflation and frequent illness in the family. The Samaritans have helped to keep me sane.'

Another woman, living unhappily with a brother, was in poor health and felt she could not cope with a move, even though her conditions were only increasing her depression. 'My brother is a miser: we have no television, phone, fridge, central heating, or car; no light in three rooms because repairs are needed and not one room has been decorated inside the house for twenty years. He insists on getting his meals first and I just have to wait every day until he has finished before starting mine, so I live mainly on casseroles which just need heating up. I found one day he was heating this for me on top of a pan of hot water, saying it took too much gas in the oven. I spend most of my time in my bedroom.'

If people lose the hope of things improving, depression quickly sets in: 'My husband has never had an interest in buying things for the home and will never pay out anything'; 'I want to get off this estate, but my husband won't move: we'll be here all my life'; 'I am so depressed in our new house that I feel I cannot go on.' One man could see no way out of his housing problems. 'The housing situation in London is appalling. No council can offer me a flat or flatlet, or even a large self-contained room. The most that is offered by accommodation agencies are tatty rooms in shabby areas at very high rents. The grim reality is that I have to live in an overcrowded guest-house, with nothing to look forward to but a dismal succession of similar places until I retire. I am sick of the vicious cycle in London of work – breakdown – work.'

Depression is often referred to as aggression turned in against the self. People who live in unsatisfactory and stressful housing conditions are, at the end of the day, more likely to gain relief from their suffering by directing their efforts towards the cause of their depression. Such forms of self-help groups as tenants' or residents' associations may, therefore, offer the most appropriate approach to their problems. If there is not a community worker in your area employed by the local authority or voluntary body, it may be useful to contact an organisation like Shelter.

FINANCIAL PROBLEMS

Financial problems may be experienced more directly by women, with a responsibility to feed and clothe a family, than by men – a fact recognised often enough by the husband: 'I know that if there is no money coming into the home, the wife just cannot cope: she has had eight years of depression.' General security is often more important to women who are particularly vulnerable, stuck at home with the children and dependent on their husbands. Domestic ties can prove a problem even to those women who do work. One young woman was joint owner of a hairdressing salon. She was faced with staff problems, combined with worry at feeling she should be at home with the children. She and her husband decided to move away and start a partnership in a new business. Her husband gave up a secure job, and she sold the salon. They then needed to remortgage the house, but failed to do so as the husband still hadn't got the new business sorted out. 'At the time I did not feel I had depression, as I seemed to be coping,' she said. 'But a few months later it hit me.' Claimants' Unions can help those on pensions and supplementary benefits.

'MID-LIFE CRISIS'

Middle age is a time of particular problems. Sayings like 'If you haven't got anywhere by the time you are forty, you never will' back up the point behind much of the depression of those years – that if you have not achieved your ambitions by then it is unlikely that you will. You are stuck with what you have made of your life, your marriage, your job, your children.

If a man or woman has failed to achieve what they wanted in their career, the prospect, at middle age, of another twenty or so years of frustration, of being stuck in a rut, is often too much to accept. It can lead to heavy drinking or gambling – an attempt to forget the future. This is liable to happen at two crisis points at work. First, if someone is not promoted at a stage when he knows he will never get another chance to attain the position he coveted. Second, if he is promoted but is promoted above his capabilities. He then worries that he will fail.

Mid-life is a time when teenage children leave home for university, distant jobs, their own flats, or get engaged or married. A woman can feel depressed enough when her child goes to nursery school, and leaves her for a short time. When the same child leaves permanently, both parents can feel a certain pointlessness in their lives, for so long dedicated to their young. Women, in particular, often have a closer, more dependent relationship with their children and at a time when they are feeling vulnerable about their own ageing they need reassurance that they are still needed.

'I realise one must learn to accept the changing pattern of one's life in the middle years,' said one woman. 'But I find myself in a position of isolation to some extent: my own children are no longer dependent on me, the rest of our families are scattered over the world, and the many friends we have made over the years live too far away to visit regularly. During my recent bout of depression, I have felt more inadequate than ever before. I feel as though, at my age, I have nothing to offer, and I have no real talents. I even panic at the thought of cooking and become utterly bewildered, ploughing through all the cookery books and recipes. I only hope that I finally come to terms with life, have my confidence restored, and have something to offer instead of this wretched feeling of despair and inadequacy.'

Women's morale is often low in these years. They have to come to terms with a different relationship, without the children; they are worried that their husbands may need to boost their own morale by getting involved with a younger woman; they are aware of getting too old to have more children (which, even if they don't want them, can have a psychological effect); and they are faced with the physical signs of the menopause.

Middle age is also a time when a severe depressive illness can occur for the first time. The clinical signs of this include marked guilt and self-reproach and paranoid delusions, occurring in someone with an obsessional personality.

However, the more common picture at this age is of mild depression. And, in the case of women, this is frequently attributed to the menopause.

MENOPAUSE

Menopause, for many years, was presented as an evil. The phrase 'It's your time of life' was used as a convenient explanation, on women from thirty to sixty-five, for every imaginable ailment from depression to headaches. Indeed, headaches, hot flushes, sweating and palpitations do occur, but they are not inevitable. Nevertheless, they naturally build up tension and depression. Menopause can start from the age of forty onwards, though menstruation does not usually cease before fifty. But fewer hormones have been produced from the ovaries for some time before that.

Certain physical changes do take place. Oestrogen, normally produced by the ovaries, is responsible for building up bones, increasing the elasticity of the skin, and nourishing the blood circulation system. It is lack of oestrogen that causes the unpleasant symptoms of the menopause. Those who suffered bad period pains in their teens are most likely to be oestrogen-deficient at the time of the menopause, and should therefore check with their doctor to see if they can be helped by oestrogen therapy.

Similar hormone therapy can be of great help in dealing premenstrual tension. Katharine Dalton's book, *Once a Month*, shows the extent to which women can suffer, and explains why this is so and what can be done about it.

But, as Dr Dalton also points out in connection with the menopausal years, 'It has been calculated that in the space of the five years around her fiftieth birthday, the average woman will lose her mother through death, her daughter through marriage and become a grandparent. There are also those whose children leave home for college or other employment, who move house or whose husband changes his job or receives his final promotion. This has led psychologists to refer to the "empty nest syndrome", believing that all the miseries of the menopausal symptoms are but a reaction to the woman's empty life.'

The problems caused by marital difficulties or children leaving home have to be faced. But physical problems associated with the menopause might well be alleviated by the use of oestrogen therapy. There are arguments for and against; but it is important to investigate any possible medical help, rather than just accept that one will remain below physical par, with the increasing depression that this will inevitably bring.

MARITAL PROBLEMS

If the central relationship on which a person has based his life begins to be eroded, it can cause a long-term depression. Sometimes, for a woman, this can start very soon after the marriage, when a man starts to batter her. Or he may constantly criticise her – a battering with words rather than fists, deliberately aimed at taking away a woman's confidence. This can reduce her to a state of numbness almost beyond depression.

In one such case, a woman of twenty-two said that she had started marriage by doing all the shopping, cooking and the financial side. 'But my husband said I wasn't capable of doing things properly. I had to pay my wages into his account and he gave me fifty pence a day to get to work and buy lunch. He got into terrible tempers; he hit me and tried to strangle me. He criticised me for untidiness and would tidy up after me: hang my clothes up, bring my nightie into me, and wait while I took my clothes off so he could put them out for washing. He went through my bag and purse, sorting out rubbish and bus tickets. He never seemed to leave me alone. He would tell me the sprouts were in too much water, that the potatoes were boiling. I have asked him to let us separate but he says he will kill me rather than let me go, and hound my parents, relations and friends. I know he would. I am so tired and listless and depressed. I don't know what to do.'

Battering, whether physical or verbal, understandably causes prolonged hopelessness. Dissatisfaction with a marriage can also cause serious depression because, again, there seems no remedy. The wife may not wish to leave because she would rather be unhappy but married than cope with living alone. Or it may be the children. One woman said, 'My true cause for depression is a very unhappy marriage, tolerated for years for the sake of my two girls, who have now grown up. Both married recently and left me, leaving me in turn with an empty life and dreadful domestic situation.'

Dr Alexandra Symonds, in her monograph *Phobias after Marriage*, says that many of her women patients, including apparently well-adjusted professional women, had one thing in common: they did not confront either themselves or their husbands with their ordinary irritation. The result, she believes, is that a phobia develops: a substitute for repressed anger.

If the cause of depression is marital disharmony and unhappiness, whether acknowledged or unacknowledged, this constitutes a long-term threat to the partner concerned, and can lead to tragic consequences, as the following case history shows.

The girl in question was young, with three children, married to a very domineering man. She had had considerable marriage problems for two or three years. Her brother tells the story:

'I went to stay with my sister over Easter one year. Six months later she was dead. The first time I realised there was something wrong was just before that Easter, when my sister rang up my mother, obviously in a state of terrible depression and desperation. She was devoted to her children and implored my mother and my wife to come up and look after them. The idea that anyone else could be asked to assist was obviously a bad sign and we arrived to find she was in a very bad state of depression. She had also become very caught up in what seemed a kind of religious fervour. It was something quite powerful in her life, which at the time seemed to her perfectly worthless.

'I found it difficult to talk to her about her belief: there was something deeply neurotic about that. It was entirely spontaneous: her husband was a stolid Church of England churchgoer, and even thumped the table and quoted the ten commandments.

'Two weeks before we came she had reached the point of knowing she needed some medical help and had gone to her GP, who had been extremely sympathetic and gave her pills, which she had not taken as she disliked drugs.

'I stayed with her for a week, but realise now that I did not make any serious attempt to discover why she was in such a bad state. Like most people, I hoped that by talking normally, the thing might go away. I remember her saying, as we got back to the house after our last drive out, "Oh, if only we could drive past, just drive on for ever." I had no idea how seriously she meant it. I returned to London the next day, leaving my wife still down there.

'At lunch the day I left, my sister had appeared to be very cheerful and had played with the children in a way she had not done for some weeks. She suggested in the afternoon that as she had a lot to do in the house, the others all went out for a walk. When they came back, they eventually found her at the top of the house: she'd taken 100 pills and a bottle of brandy and was lying on the bed that she had prepared as a last resting-place. She had been so cunning about it – managing to get them all out of the way, and to have my wife there to look after the children if she vanished, as she wanted to do.

'She was taken to an intensive care unit and after three days she was brought to the point where she was obviously going to recover. She then seemed, for a few days, much more cheerful again. She got on very well with the nurse in the unit and thought lucidly in a way she had not been doing with the family – although she had no sympathy with the psychiatrist, who in turn had no sympathy with her. She obviously could not stay indefinitely in the unit, and it was the psychiatrist's view that she had to be signed off and sent home.

'But her reason for not wanting to live was the situation at home. She had become deeply disenchanted with her husband, and had been having an affair with someone else. The make-up of her husband, in conjunction with her own, was disastrous. Sometimes people seem to pick out someone who is going to bring out the worst in them. My sister had reached the point of coming up against a brick wall, because of her commitment to her children. She knew that if she went off with another man she would lose the custody of the children. And so she had got to the stage of wanting to kill herself. She wanted to get out of the situation she was in, into some new life with her children, and she couldn't see any way of doing it.

'When she was in the intensive care unit, the only visitor allowed was her husband – and she didn't want to see him. But she found it impossible to say to his face that she wanted to get away from him.

'She begged a close friend not to let them send her home to her husband. We found it enormously difficult talking to the husband about what should be done as he was blind to the problem. All he wanted to know was that she loved him and admired him and wanted to come home – and that she seemed to be well enough to do so. The first thing he said to her when he saw her in the intensive care unit was, "It's all right, I have brought my book." This was one he'd written. And after he saw her the next time he said to us: "She's much better, she's read my book." At the same time, she said to her friend, "He's brought in that dreadful book." It was complete non-communication between the two people most involved.

'The husband wanted her home but we eventually prevailed upon him to send her to a nursing home. It proved disastrous. Despite its expense, there were no qualified nursing staff. One day the doctor said she was to have ECT treatment, about which she had very strong views. Late that night, an orderly said, "Your ECT is tomorrow, you just have to sign this form." She left it with my sister, who then took a light bulb out of the socket and scored her wrists, as a protest. The doctor considered his professional authority was being called into question and that if she would not follow his recommendation to have ECT there was no point in her remaining there.

'There was then a family conference about where she should go, and she went to a large hospital in a university town. She was under two psychiatrists, neither of whom she took to. One of these told her, "There is nothing wrong with you, you have made an exhibition of yourself, you have got to go home and face up to your problems." She said that she didn't want to go home; that it was the only place she *didn't* want to go. And that she really wanted to go back to the intensive care unit, where she had received more understanding.

'The same psychiatrist sent word to her that the following day she was going to be discharged and her husband would pick her up. She went out with some friends for an hour that day and was very depressed, though she did not tell them she was going to be discharged. When they took her back, they looked for someone to warn that she was depressed, but couldn't find anyone, so went away. The next morning she was found in the lavatory. She had hanged herself.'

At the inquest, one of the psychiatrists said that she had not been considered a suicide risk, and that it must have been due to something which happened during the night, or when out with her friends. The brother felt very strongly that the psychiatrists had been totally unsympathetic to her depression and made no attempt to find out its cause.

In a rather similar case, a woman who had a great deal of stress in her married life – basically through having to work long hours and cope with all family decisions and finance because of an inadequate husband, who relied on drink – finally attempted suicide. She was hardly even aware of being depressed, having become gradually more and more remote and distanced from life. She was sent to a psychiatric hospital, where she was kept under heavy sedation for several weeks. There was, again, no attempt to investigate her problems and she still felt too remote from it all to talk much about it. After another week or so, the psychiatrist decided she could be discharged. She was rapidly taken off the major drugs she was on, which left her feeling very shaky. She went home and, the same night, made another suicide attempt.

Worried about a repeat performance at the hospital, her doctor gambled and suggested she joined the household of a therapeutic healer who had been successful in helping people overcome severe depression before. There was no laid-down treatment as such: she was taken off drugs; made to work physically hard in the house; sent for long walks; not allowed to see her husband or children, though she could see certain members of her family, and could talk over any problems with the healer. He also talked to the husband. After six months, he told her she could go and stay with her friends, though must not go home yet. Three months later, he suggested she took a part-time job, while staying with a member of her family, in order to build up her confidence. It was only at that time that the drugs she had been given in hospital were really getting out of her system. Ultimately she returned to her husband and children, and has coped adequately since then.

TREATMENT

Different types of treatment in use for depression are listed in Appendix I. What follows here is an account of experiences people have had with treatment: what *is* on offer as opposed to what should be on offer. And why, with them, it has or has not worked.

Faced with a person who is showing signs of anxiety, stress or mild depression, doctors often prescribe psychotropic drugs – that is, tranquillisers, sedatives and antidepressants. These drugs were developed in the 1950s and have proved a major breakthrough in controlling symptoms of mental illness, and have dramatically reduced the average length of time that patients spend in psychiatric hospitals.

But family doctors now prescribe 3,000 million of these psychotropic drugs a year in Britain. They are regarded as a panacea and are prescribed, or asked for, for even minor upsets. Many people are aware of their increasing dependence on them and would like to come off them – but do not know what else to do.

Listening to depressed people you hear the same remarks about drugs time and time again: 'I have been put on all the latest antidepressants, but they numb my brain and I don't know what I'm doing half the time'; 'I have been taking tranquillisers for four years; they help for a time, but then I cry and feel choked'; 'I can cope if I take the tablets, but hate to feel that I can only live some normal life with these drugs'; 'I have no faith at all in all these drugs, but without them, what is there?'

It may be that the treatment prescribed by doctor or psychiatrist entails long-term use of antidepressants. But this should be checked out with them. Do not just ask the receptionist for a repeat prescription. Go in and see your medical practitioner, so that *he* can see how you are responding to the drug and whether you need a repeat or possibly some other form of treatment.

The other main complaint has been about the side-effects of

prescribed tranquillisers and antidepressants (*these are listed more fully in Appendix I*). When the National Association for Mental Health's magazine, *Mind Out*, ran a special issue on psychiatry, asking for readers' complaints, it received trenchant criticisms about the effects of drugs. 'Although the antidepressants control the worst attacks of uncontrollable weeping and accompanying feelings of utter despair, they do not lift the depression and they leave my wife devoid of interest in her normal activities and unable to think properly,' said one man. But much of the criticism was concentrated on the lack of information from doctors when they hand out drugs, and the lack of notice they seem to take of patients' complaints of side-effects. One woman said, 'Often the side effects are damaging and can cause a personality change that destroys family relationships.'

Another patient, who was transferred from drug to drug to deal with her depression, was entirely ignorant of the side-effects of these drugs. The lack of information led her to increase the dosage when she felt the drugs were not helping. The next morning, she was unable to speak and could not swallow. One patient wrote: 'Why can't doctors treat patients as intelligent people who want to know what the diagnosis is, how the pills are to benefit, what their side-effects are and what would happen if they don't take them – or take too many? Or have alcohol?'

Many doctors and psychiatrists are aware of this criticism. One north London doctor found that his own patients benefited greatly from about six 'talking treatment' sessions with him, backed up by a course of drugs. 'We should never think of drugs as the whole answer,' he said. 'But at a time of acute mental stress, they can be useful in relieving that stress, so that the underlying symptoms can then be treated. They act as a sort of crutch, but they must be supervised closely.' And a consultant psychiatrist said, 'Before you accept drug treatment, it should be sold to you. Drugs may be an essential part of your treatment. But if the doctor cannot explain why, go to someone else.'

At a conference on 'The Uses and Limitations of Psychotropic Drugs in General Practice', held at the Royal Society of Medicine, one psychiatrist said: 'When I deal with a patient who I think will be a resistant depressive, I provide them with a small written document. The first point mentioned on this is the name of the drug given to them, followed by explicit instructions: for instance, one tablet three times a day until Saturday, and then two tablets three times a day thereafter. I tell them to come and see me twice a week, also that they can expect side-effects. I tell them not to stop taking the tablets without consulting me and, lastly, not to expect these tablets to act for at least two weeks and probably longer.'

Patients are often unaware of this time-lag and naturally expect some encouraging reaction to the drug within a few days. A survey, reported at the conference, found that nearly 60 per cent of patients in group general practices had stopped taking their tricyclic drugs before the end of the third week, and nearly 70 per cent before reaching the fourth week – which is when it can be judged if the drug is working. Of the remainder, only half were taking the drugs consistently.

The same survey also found that only 7 per cent of patients stopped their drugs because of the side-effects – normally regarded as the reason. In fact, other explanations were given: the prescription ran out; they thought the drugs had not helped them much, anyway; they believed they were beginning to get better and now was the time to stop.

Another reason why depressed people do not follow instructions is simply that they are already in an unhappy and bewildered mental state and their concentration and memory may well be poor. They are often also drowsy – sometimes as a result of the drugs, sometimes because of their depressed condition – and relatives frequently refrain from giving the patient the full dose because they think it too strong for someone who seems half-drugged already.

It is worth checking with the doctor or psychiatrist to see if a dose given, perhaps, three times a day cannot be given in its entirety at night – which might get over some of the difficulties of side-effects and also help the disturbed sleep often experienced by depressives.

Many people feel they cannot cope with continuing unhappiness without the boost of pills. Tranquillisers or antidepressants can, indeed, successfully help someone over a crisis by calming them, preventing constant tears, giving them an ability to cope for the time being. But as a psychiatrist at the medical conference pointed out: 'There is a myth, generated by us and by pharmaceutical firms, as well as by patients, that unhappiness and anxiety should not be endured and are treatable by pharmacological means. A most useful function all of us can perform is to tell people the truth: that there is anxiety and unhappiness and that these are not really amenable to treatment by pharmacological means. Certainly, as a consultant psychiatrist, I see people who are suffering anxiety or unhappiness quite appropriate to their situation and their personality. We do people a disservice if they are started off on this chain of pharmacological treatment.'

It is important that people are told that their depression may be quite normal, given their circumstances. Some depressives I spoke to, or heard from, had had disastrous experiences that understandably could take years to get over. If they had, for instance, nursed a sick parent who subsequently died, they naturally suffered from both the loss of the parent and the sudden lack of meaning in their life. They may, indeed, never come to terms with this. And many believe that it is the job of pills to help them do so. As another doctor said: 'So often patients come in after bereavement and ask for something for a week or two to "tide them over" after the loss of a loved one. It is tempting to give them a tranquilliser for a week. At the end of a week they return, saying they are not quite over it yet. Before you know what has happened, the weeks slip by and they have been on tranquillisers for months.'

Many people nowadays are finding themselves less able to accept their normal reaction to bereavement, or their normal distress under upsetting circumstances. But drugs, taken to dampen down reality, become less and less effective and ultimately bring the additional problems of side-effects. They are not, as many people painfully find out, the universal solution. Only those judged as having a chemical inbalance may have to depend on drugs, long-term, to function.

ELECTROCONVULSIVE THERAPY (ECT)

If, after some four weeks, a patient does not respond to the more powerful antidepressants, the doctor may refer him to a psychiatrist.

The psychiatrist will see the patient, review the treatment, and may suggest an alternative. In a minority of cases, this is ECT treatment.

ECT (*see also Appendix I*) is a very emotive subject. It is more frequently used to treat depression than any other mental illness, and its results have often been dramatic. One psychiatrist, working in a hospital in 1941, when ECT was introduced there, said he could hardly believe the effect on the rows of chronically depressed patients in the wards, for whom there had been no real treatment. 'But on the introduction of ECT they got better and went home. It was stamped on my memory.'

Reactions from the depressives I spoke to varied greatly. Some praised it, looked upon it as a life-saver, and had no qualms about having it again. Others complained of loss of memory after the treatment. One young girl in her early twenties who spent a year in a psychiatric hospital and had several ECT treatments said: 'I was told my memory would come back, but it never has properly. Sometimes my mother will look back at old snapshot albums, and I can see pictures of myself on the beach, so I know I was there. But I can't remember it.' Others said they had been anxious to try this treatment because they felt so ill that anything was worth trying. With some it had worked well and they were quite prepared to have it again if they relapsed; some said that it simply had not done much good.

There are a lot of upsetting stories about ECT and more of these tend to be passed on than the good experiences which patients recall. One man, for example, said that he had a course of sixteen ECTs, at the rate of two a week. 'The waiting-room was bright and there were flowers in the room; there were books to read and music to listen to. We had to lie on a trolley, when it was our turn, with a red blanket to cover us. There is nothing to be frightened about: the anaesthetic was Pentothal and a wonderful feeling comes over one before losing consciousness. The next thing I knew was waking up in another room with a cup of tea waiting.'

There is no point in chronicling the upsetting experiences – though Chapter 9 on patients' rights contains some important warnings in this connection – because many people may only become unnecessarily worried if ECT should be prescribed for them or a relative. The necessity for this treatment, however, should be discussed with the psychiatrist. Dr Anthony Clare, in his book *Psychiatry in Dissent*, does not condemn its use, but stresses that treatment involving an anaesthetic and muscle relaxant is hardly a trivial procedure and that it is far easier for a psychiatrist to recommend a course of ECT than to carry out psychotherapy in depth. ECT, he feels, is therefore a 'much abused and over-used method of treatment.'

Why ECT works, when it works, is not known. But as one university lecturer in mental health told me: 'ECT can be very relevant with desperate and suffering people. It can transform a person and get him to a point when he can begin to apply himself to his problems. But although it can improve you a lot, and make you able to cope with life, it isn't the answer: drugs and ECT don't actually solve the problems.'

GROUP THERAPY

One way of tackling problems of depression is group therapy – used in psychiatric hospitals for both in-patients and out-patients. It is particularly aimed at helping people with difficulties in personal relationships or with communication. The group is guided by a therapist, but it is meant to provide an opportunity for members to air and discuss their thoughts and problems.

'I went for five days a week,' said one man of about forty, who had been an in-patient at the time. 'We were all of a type; all from the same background with the same symptoms of depression. We all seemed to have suffered a loss of parent in some sense, either as an evacuee, or because of their divorce. There were a lot of incidents that we had all suppressed. I knew that I was not alone, that the others felt the same – even though, to me, my alienation was special. The group opened me up a lot. We mostly talked. Some days you sit in the group and think 'What a load of rubbish'. Other days you are alert and caring.

'In the group, you either shut up or you act in front of everyone. I reacted to people through the topic. You do build up relationships in time within the group and you do actually care and look out for each other. I think for me that form of treatment was probably the better kind. I think that ECT can put you back on your feet, but it doesn't give you that reservoir of information to work with in the future.'

The average length of treatment with group psychotherapy is from eighteen months to two years; and members attending for such a length of time obviously form a close-knit group. One girl being treated for depression in a psychiatric hospital said: 'The group had been going for some time when I joined and they were all very close. The first time I went there I felt like an outsider. They all questioned me, but I did not know a thing about them and I just wanted to run away. One girl, I felt, really did not want me there. She had a cushion, and she made out it was this guy she blamed, and she was lashing into it. I just didn't feel part of it.'

Dr Brian Wijesinghe, Principal Psychologist of Claybury Hospital, says that when a person has a generalised depression, feels lethargic and pessimistic and has very little interest in what is going on he finds the best approach is either individual psychotherapy – allowing the patient to talk through to the underlying reasons for his depression – or group psychotherapy. 'Some people are much more able to accept the idea that others with similar problems are in a position to help them; that they will not expect an expert or all-knowing doctor to solve all their problems; and that they must take major responsibility for their own problems and put some effort into trying to work through their difficulties. Patients who are more authority-minded, and want a doctor to solve their problems, are quite reluctant to accept group therapy and, even after several months or even years, they change very little. People who have positive expectations about a certain treatment are more likely to accept it and find it provides an answer to their problems. It's quite an important factor in the treatment of emotionally disturbed patients.'

As well as individual and group psychotherapy, those with depression try every manner of help on offer, often in desperation. Some have found that acupuncture, in which the body and mind are treated as a whole, is of some success; some try hypnotherapy – where the patient is helped to relax and, when in this relaxed mood, is more open to talking about what may have caused the depression and to suggestions about practical ways of coping. Marriage guidance counsellors also have a great deal of experience in helping with relationship problems; and the British Association of Counsellors has a membership list of trained counsellors who can listen and guide people.

DIET

There is growing awareness that eliminating certain foods from one's diet can have a direct bearing on mental health. This idea is still far from being generally accepted, despite the evidence of recovery in some apparently intractable cases. As Dr Richard Mackarness says in his book *Not all in the Mind*, 'It is easy to accept as allergic the rash which appears when a susceptible person eats shellfish or strawberries but harder to recognise that the bread or eggs he eats every day may be causing his bouts of catarrh, headache and mental depression.' In one of the cases he treated, a woman who suffered from nasal allergy, fatigue and disabling mental depression said she found it a wonderful relief to know that her 'tiredness and miserable self-accusation' could be switched off if she stopped eating eggs and milk.

For those interested in the dietary approach – and many have welcomed it as a breakthrough – tests and procedures are given in Dr Mackarness's book. He warns, however, that these should only be carried out with your doctor's approval and co-operation.

THE NEED TO TALK

Depressives have an overwhelming need to talk to someone – except for those whose depression is so severe that they have become remote and withdrawn from the world. Many undoubtedly find it hard to talk to their partner, parents, or nearest relations, because it may be those very people whose actions or behaviour are at the root of the depression. But the need to talk remains.

'I have felt so alone that it has become unbearable to go on living,' said one woman. 'I have cried and prayed for someone, anyone, to talk to. That was the hardest part to bear. Although my doctor was marvellous when I had a physical illness requiring an operation and after-care, he just didn't have the time to listen when I was depressed, and help talk it through.' Another said: 'If only I could talk to someone who really understands and to be able to talk and talk and talk – without the feeling of obligation or fear of taking up too much of their time. I feel strongly that so much is still bottled up inside me, wanting to come out, despite having had an awful lot of psychiatric treatment, two quite long spells in the local psychiatric hospital, including ECT, and also having two suicide attempts behind me. I've had a very long and bitter struggle to overcome very deep depression and the suppression of feelings and rejection that I know caused it.'

Many depressed people are very aware that they themselves cannot make much effort to meet people who might help them – 'the most difficult thing to do is to join clubs and various organised activities' – and stress they want to talk to someone who understands their feelings. As one said, 'I need to talk to people who have suffered depression in order that I can gauge how far up the ladder of recovery I have progressed and just how much I must accept as my own personality, defects and failings.'

Another unmarried young mother said that she found she could not talk to people in authority, like her doctor, social worker or probation officer; neither had she any friends to talk to. Her depression was such that she dreaded to think what would happen to her baby. One woman, who phoned the Samaritans when in particular despair, said that her greatest help 'was talking to someone who had no personal contact with me, who would talk, but not insist that *this* was what I needed, or *that*, but would just listen.'

Depressed people are very conscious that others get exasperated with their apparent failure to make any attempt to counteract depression. Their wish to talk to those who have gone through depression is because they are aware that only depressives can begin to understand how they feel.

LACK OF UNDERSTANDING

One woman, endorsing this, said: 'I am practically cut off. I find that my husband and daughter lack understanding. It's such a dreadful illness and it just goes on and on. I feel very bitter as I used to be so active and never asked for any help in the house at all. Nothing was too much trouble, but all I can do now is essentials. I just sit staring into space.' A man of sixty-one said: 'From my teenage days I have suffered so much from depression, and this is something most people do not understand. You can't seem to explain the terrible feeling you are having while all the while trying to appear normal and OK. How can you tell someone you are scared of losing your reason, when they think so much of you, nominating you for committees and looking up to you as a steadying influence on everything? I know I upset my wife and family sometimes, but I just can't tell them how I feel.' His reaction was similar to that of another woman: 'My immediate family don't seem to know how terrible this illness is. To them it is a depression like everyone gets from time to time.'

Another man of thirty-two, who had been depressed for nearly five years and has been on sickness benefit for twelve months, said that he did not think that 'doctors and others realise the despair and helplessness one feels. I know some people can pull themselves together, as they say, but others of us cannot. I have had every treatment, including ECT, but live on edge that my benefit will be stopped because they do not class depression as an illness. I know it is crippling for anyone to be depressed severely, but for a young man like myself it is heartbreaking to be treated like a malingerer.'

SUPPORT GROUPS

The value of personal support, whether through a friend or group, cannot be overestimated at a time when your own opinion of yourself and your ability to cope is at a low ebb. It is important to make contact with, or set up, a survival network in advance, at a time when you are feeling mentally able to cope. Otherwise, when you need this help, you may feel too remote or despairing to organise anything.

A small group of people who have been through the same experience as yourself can be particularly helpful. By contacting such a group in advance you can telephone or write or ask a group member to visit you when you need help.

One such group is Depressives Anonymous. This has been running for five years and there is now a network of about twenty groups in Britain. Its aim is to provide reassurance, motivation and constant encouragement. In no way does the organisation oppose the professional treatment of depression; it is anxious to work in tandem whenever possible. It hopes that doctors and hospitals will advise patients to contact any of its groups when other methods seem to be failing, or 'recovered' patients need support or help in following up whatever form of therapy is needed to help them function again.

In talking about Depressives Anonymous, Keith Middleton, the chairman, gives a list of similarities present in most depressive experiences: isolation, inadequacy, indecision, exaggeration of problems, fear of intellectual impairment, lack of understanding, lack of communication, lack of concentration, fatigue, lapses of memory. He suggests those with depression write down their own thoughts and emotions under each heading, repeating this at different times, possibly when there is a change of mood. This he believes, is the way to understanding and developing an attitude of mind towards individual depression. Contact with a fellow sufferer in a mutual support group, or by post, encourages the comparison and sharing of the problems and difficulties of depression.

Everyone involved in Depressives Anonymous is either a present or past sufferer from depression, as a fundamental belief of the organisation is self-help and mutual help. This giving as well as taking is important: an active helper in July may be in desperate need of help in August. As most depressives go through a period of searching for some reason for their condition, helping others similarly placed helps provide some purpose.

Most Depressives Anonymous contacts do not wish to become permanent members of a group. DA aims at personal, supporting relationships between fellow sufferers, each having two or more contacts – telephone numbers and addresses – with whom they feel easy and relaxed. The group's meetings exist for those who want them – to introduce new contacts. No one is made to feel guilty if he does not attend, or is not in touch, as it is presumed that support is not needed at that time.

Another such group is Depressives Associated. Janet Stevenson started Depressives Associated some six years ago – claiming that, during her own depression, she encountered a lack of understanding and tolerance from those around her, particularly from the medical profession, to whom she still feels hostile. She stresses the importance of becoming involved in non-domestic interests and continuing intellectual activity. Anyone interested is asked to become a group organiser. Six newsletters a year are sent to members and there is a membership fee.

MIND

The National Association for Mental Health (MIND) has a number of local associations throughout the country. Those with mental ill-health – as well as their relatives or partners – can go there for advice, or to meet others similarly placed. Some of these associations have also set up mental health facilities in areas where services are poor. Blackburn and Lancaster MIND associations, for example, both run vigorous counselling centres and, late in 1979, Liverpool MIND opened the first mental health resource centre in the north-west.

PRACTICAL SUGGESTIONS

1 Certain drugs may need to be taken long-term, or during cycles of depression until these episodes are over. Others are needed as mood stabilisers over a shorter period of crisis which has arisen through circumstances. Drugs should be taken long-term only on the advice of doctor or psychiatrist, and you or a relative should check with either or both of these that your condition requires long-term treatment and how long it is likely to be.

If you have asked for drugs to help over a crisis, at a time when you cannot function without such help, you should see the doctor each time you want a renewed prescription. In these circumstances drugs can only blanket your mind from the cause of depression: they cannot be expected to cure the cause itself.

2 For certain kinds of depression, drug treatment is the best

treatment. But check with your doctor or psychiatrist whether this is so in your case, or whether any other kind of treatment (such as psychotherapy) is a genuine alternative.

3   If the cause is circumstances, such as bereavement or loss of some kind, or environmental, it may be that you can make an appointment with your doctor to have a longer talk about it, or that there is some counselling support available as part of the general practice team. Otherwise, ask the doctor if he knows of any local counselling support. Marriage guidance counsellors, for example, despite their name, counsel in areas like bereavement and separation or divorce. If your doctor is unable to help, ask any local advice centre, or write to the appropriate psychotherapy or counselling addresses, or MIND.

4   Support is often needed at times when depression, for no apparent reason, seems to worsen. It is usually possible for you, or a relation or friend, to be aware of the signs that these blacker periods are starting. Contact with a support group (*see under this heading*) is of particular importance here – by phone or letter, if you feel unable to go to a meeting.

Setting up a mutual survival network with a particular friend is another, or supplementary, method. It needs to be someone who has also experienced depression, who fully understands the situation and who you, in turn, can help when necessary.

5   After leaving psychiatric hospital for treatment for depression, you will normally attend as an out-patient. You or your relatives should ask about day-centre facilities, or any other after-care facilities run by the hospital. Ask in particular if there is any crisis intervention service run by the hospital (sometimes there may be a local service, unattached to the hospital). The aim of such a service is to provide support to you and your family in any emergency, with the hope of keeping you out of a further – or indeed initial – period in hospital. There is a danger that constant admission to psychiatric hospital breeds 'career patients'.

In addition, ask the hospital whether there is a community psychiatric nurse who is contactable in an emergency, or can generally monitor your progress if you fear being unable to cope on your own. Any social worker with whom you are in touch will be told by the hospital that you have left, and can also visit and provide support.

6 If you have a desperate need to talk urgently, telephone the Samaritans, who also run a befriending service, in which a person is appointed to visit and support you.

7 Getting a job may be difficult after any psychiatric treatment. For advice on this, see the '*Employment*' section in Chapter 9.

8 For some people, depression is caused by specific happenings – as with, for example, prisoners' wives or those who are disabled. Here specific organisations may be of help (*see Appendix II*). With depression at polytechnics or universities, the resident counsellor is likely to be experienced in the problems which arise.

9 If you are a friend, colleague, or relation of the person who is depressed it is important to offer as much support as you are able, either at the beginning (when you may be needed to go to the doctor with the person), or during any other time of obvious stress. A person's presence alone can sometimes help, even if no gratitude is expressed.

GENERAL COMMENTS ON RECOVERY

Sometimes, quite minor involvement can help. A Scotswoman said that she had got a voluntary job for just two hours a day – all she felt she could manage – and that 'I know now that getting involved in something outside the family is the answer to my basic feelings of inadequacy.' Another who took a job involving repetition and organisation said she found it was the only way to calm her chaotic mind. One middle-aged woman, whose children had left home, said that she had started going to church and 'met some wonderful people. I seem to be able to talk to them and it helps to know you're useful to someone.' And a man was helped when he became a counter-hand at a small corner shop, as 'listening to the problems the shoppers had lifted my own depression'.

Those who can manage to get out to any kind of social club or gathering – such as clubs aimed at divorced or separated people, Darby and Joan clubs, day centres – have often been helped by their new contacts. One man said that the most therapeutic setting for him was the launderette. Some elderly women who feel isolated and depressed have been helped by the constructive 'Adopt a Granny' scheme An 'adopted granny' may provide invaluable help and support to a family, while at the same time gaining a great deal for herself. One person told me, 'We were approached by a health visitor concerning an elderly retired midwife, who was very depressed and lonely. We needed a baby-sitter and she needed company and some purpose in her life. Our needs very much complemented one another, and now she is a very valued member of our family.'

Another woman said that she did not feel like going out, 'but I find that painting is a wonderful help, for one cannot worry and paint; it needs all the concentration possible'. Another bought a puppy, which made her feel 'as if I were coming out of a dark tunnel'.

Sometimes, the effort of accomplishing anything practical needs the support of family or friends, despite the emotional battering that these, too, are probably going through. One woman said that one of the main factors in her recovery, medication and a good psychiatrist apart, had been the support of her family, 'especially in the form of my children's unerring respect and unbelievable outspoken love', which helped her build up her self-respect. Another was helped by her husband throwing all her pills down the lavatory when he realised what a zombie she had become ('At least I knew he cared').

One young wife said that, two weeks after being discharged from hospital, after an overdose, she had been lying in bed when her best friend had called. 'She rang the bell twice, but I didn't bother answering. Anyway, the house was so dirty, and untidy, that even in the state I was in I was a little ashamed of it. My friend had a key to our house and she came upstairs and said, "Get up, we're going out, I'm sick of seeing your husband having to cook his own meals and wash his own clothes, and yours." She went on to say that my husband was seriously considering walking out on me and that my mother was making herself ill with worry. I was too listless to argue. I got up, dressed and we went shopping, then sat and talked. My friend never again mentioned my behaviour or my state of mind. She chattered on and on about people we knew, places we'd been, things we'd done. I began to relax and, when my husband arrived home that night, his dinner was in the oven and I was in a brand-new dress. His pleasure made the expense worthwhile. My friend came every single day, weekends included, for about six months. Gradually she cut down her visits until I knew that I could and would cope alone. I realise that she had confidence in herself to enable her to give me self-confidence.

'Not long after, she lost her husband in a tragic accident. She was pregnant, but her experience with my depression stopped her from breaking down. Once again, we saw each other frequently, and this time I was able to help her.'

Depression is a way of withdrawing from life. People's personality, upbringing or constitution may predispose them towards depression, but it is usually triggered off by circumstances. And this may require some difficult decisions about either accepting the situation or taking steps to change it – before the inertia associated with depression sets in and renders any decision or course of action impossible.

The earlier depression is noticed, by a relation or colleague if not by the sufferer, the easier it is to treat – by whatever method. It is important to remember that support is always available from some source. It is equally important to remember that some 60 per cent of those with depression get well spontaneously in time.

6

Post-natal Depression

'I am just beginning to get over an attack of post-natal depression and, for me, it was like the end of the world,' said a young mother of nearly twenty, after the birth of her first baby. When she had arrived home from hospital, she had felt rather low in spirits for a week or so. Gradually, her depression worsened. 'In the end, I could not eat anything because of my nerves,' she said, 'and this was depressing me more.' Her doctor gave her antidepressants and tried to reassure her that the depression would pass. But for months she went to doctor after doctor, trying to get confirmation that there was nothing seriously wrong with her mentally.

Most expectant mothers know of the term 'post-natal depression', but as it is often mistakenly used to describe any kind of emotional disturbance after birth many of these mothers still do not know what to expect.

Post-natal emotional disturbance falls, in fact, into three main categories.

First, *post partum blues* (*post partum* means 'after birth'). These are popularly called 'three-day blues' and are very common: some four-fifths of mothers experience them. They are transient feelings of mild or quite intense depression, occurring within three days or so of delivery.

Second, *post-natal depression*. A much smaller proportion of women find that they are depressed for a longer period – a few weeks or months, even for some years.

Third, *puerperal psychosis*. This affects a very small number of women – perhaps one or two in every 1,000 confinements. It is mental illness which begins during the puerperium (the period of labour and shortly after) and is apparently connected with, or precipitated by, childbirth or motherhood. The degree of severity generally necessitates admission to hospital.

The cause of the first category, *three-day blues*, is unknown, or at least unproved. Theories include hormone changes (such as the massive drop in the level of progesterone after the birth), the replacement of anticipation by reality, the reaction to the physical shock of having a baby, and breast-feeding problems.

The National Childbirth Trust, founded to improve women's knowledge about childbirth, holds antenatal classes in many parts of the country. In its teaching, it tries to prepare pregnant women for these see-saw emotions and the short time they last, because when these emotions are expected they are easier to accept.

What is less easy for a new mother to accept is to find herself suffering from the more prolonged *post-natal depression*, rather than the three-day blues.

Post-natal depression comes as a particular shock to a new mother, as motherhood is invariably portrayed as the height of happiness. Television mothers can be seen beaming away as they choose the right washing powder for the nappies; women's magazine covers portray gurgling babies hugged by happy wives. The depressed mother cannot understand why she feels as she does, so added to her depression are feelings of shame and guilt and a reluctance to admit her despair.

The husband is also not necessarily of much help here, as he too has expected the child's birth to be a time of happiness. One woman wrote in *Nursing Mirror*: 'The change from a happy, expectant woman looking forward only to the birth of her baby, to a depressed and weeping mother – who, once she has returned home, is so tired she feels she cannot cope and, consequently, that the baby is nothing but a nuisance – is a great emotional shock to the husband.'

This particular woman attributed her depression to the way things were handled after the birth. First, the baby was placed in a cot on the side of the delivery room where she could not see him or touch him when he whimpered. This may seem a minor matter, but the new mother's emotions are very sensitive at that time. Second, the baby had been born in the late afternoon and the mother went to sleep. On waking, she found the baby was in the night nursery and she couldn't see him until the next morning: 'Even now, ten months later, it upsets me to think of the way I was parted from him so soon after birth.' Third, no one explained to her the technique of breast-feeding; and she was also upset at having to wait for the routine feeding times because, before then, the baby would be crying from hunger.

Admitting her depression only worsened matters: 'Part of my treatment was the enforced periods of rest when my baby was taken away from me. This only increased my depression and also gave me a strong sense of failure. I felt I was incapable of looking after him.'

The events surrounding the birth, and of the birth itself, are of major importance in determining whether or not post-natal depression occurs.

Jean Robinson, who was at one time Chairman of the Patients' Association, told me that she had received many letters from women about childbirth experiences and that she was surprised how often stories of unkind treatment during labour were correlated with depression. Many mothers become extremely anxious after having to submit to painful procedures and, in cases of extreme pain after some induced labours, relive the experience for months or years after. Those not fully awake at the time of birth, due to the drugs administered, said that their feeling for the baby was affected. The same lack of feeling occurred if the baby was taken away before the mother had a chance to hold him.

In *Some Mothers' Experience of Induced Labour*, an investigation into the experiences of induced births by the National Childbirth Trust, compiled by Sheila Kitzinger, it was found that the mother and infant were frequently separated after the induction. The mothers of the induced babies had their attitude to the babies affected by this separation. As one said: 'The baby appeared to react violently against me when he met me eventually and against breast-feeding attempts ... only gradually could I "unfreeze" towards him inside.' She went on to say that she had remained 'detached' from the baby for about a year.

Other mothers who later suffered from post-natal depression

had similar upsetting experiences. Particularly mentioned was their wish to touch the baby, which had been refused on the grounds that it was time for it to be washed, put under a heater, weighed, and so on. This enforced and often unnecessary separation from their infants can seriously jeopardise the mother's feelings of attachment towards their children.

Certain other birth experiences can also foster detachment. A mother, quoted in the report, who was given epidural anaesthesia (an injection into the spinal column which numbs the lower part of the body) said, 'I felt terribly detached watching in the mirror, and a little guilty because I felt that everybody expected me to be over-whelmed with joy.' Later, she suffered from post-natal depression for several months.

Another said: 'If I had not woken as the baby was being born, I would never have believed him mine.' This feeling persisted with one mother and merged into depression: 'I find myself going to pieces, withdrawn into myself.' She then described how she found herself hitting the baby without reason and became very frightened.

Apart from experiences at the time of giving birth, social factors can play a part in the onset of post-natal depression. George Brown and Tirril Harris, in *Social Origins of Depression*, found that out of twelve depressed patients, with either a birth or a pregnancy during a year, five were living in grossly inadequate housing, five had very bad marriages where continued support for the new child was called into question, one was an unmarried girl who later had an abortion, and one involved a later miscarriage. They consider that the result shows that pregnancy and birth, like other crises, can bring home to a woman the hopelessness of her position; or make her feel even more dependent on an uncertain relationship.

Janet Stevenson, who runs Depressives Associated, believes that post-natal depression is a change-of-gear breakdown. 'So many girls now do not learn the basic homekeeping chores, and have very little to do with babies. When they discover that their babies are not little dolls, but real live demanding individuals, then their confidence evaporates and a depression starts.' Another reason, in her opinion, for the onset of depression is that women who previous to the birth, had a stimulating or busy job, find that being a mother, with its humdrum routine, brings on depression: 'stimulation, not tranquillisation, may answer some of the problems of young mothers' depression.'

The very small percentage of mothers who suffer from the third category, *puerperal psychosis*, may have had previous mental illness. The birth triggers off a depressive illness or mania. One girl, for instance, who had had bouts of agitated excitement in the past, became very elated on becoming a mother. But her elation spiralled so high that, according to one friend, 'she went over the top'. She was admitted to a psychiatric hospital and, for a week or so, had severe mood swings, alternatively wanting to hug the baby and then becoming depressed and expressing total lack of interest in it. Although she finally improved, under drug treatment, the same thing happened when she had her second child. This time she spent longer in hospital, and her doctor advised her not to have a third child.

Treatment for puerperal psychosis is usually undertaken in hospital. But if treatment is at home it is better for the family helpers to help the mother care for the baby, rather than remove it from her. There is a risk, however, that the mother's mental state could result in her harming the child.

PRACTICAL MEASURES

The National Childbirth Trust holds antenatal classes in many parts of the country, which prepare women physically and psychologically for childbirth, and form the basis of a post-natal support system. The Trust provides breast-feeding counsellors who visit homes and postnatal support workers who will also visit and discuss any problems which have arisen. It also provides a counselling service on all nonmedical problems connected with childbirth. It has over eighty local groups which offer social activities and companionship to mothers who feel isolated and insecure.

Involving the father at the outset (by, for example, his presence at the delivery) is important both psychologically and practically. If he can get paternity leave or even take part of his annual leave right after the birth, and share the burden of chores like changing nappies and cooking, it will halve the mother's tiredness and also involve the father with the child. With the first child, in particular, there is a need to adjust to being a family, no longer a couple.

When a new mother first arrives home from hospital, she needs immediate support – preferably by getting in a grandmother, mother or mother-in-law to help – in fact, anyone who can offer practical and moral support.

Having a background of advice from antenatal classes is important at this stage. One mother, for example, was particularly helped because it had been stressed at these classes that feelings of closeness to the baby may well not come for several weeks.

Midwives and health visitors also provide practical advice and information. One young mother said that she had only coped on her return home because the health visitor established a feeding pattern and daily routine, interspersed with rest periods. 'This greatly reduced my sense of muddle-headedness. I was so tired when I returned home from hospital that even pegging out the nappies on the line seemed a major chore I could not face.'

Physical fatigue plays a large part in reducing a mother's mental ability to cope – a fact often unrecognised by new mothers, whose feelings about their mind and body are divorced. (Inducing fatigue is a well-known technique used in brainwashing, to cause disorientation.) It is usually impossible to get a good night's sleep when a baby has to be fed in the night, but any chance to catnap during the day, when the baby is asleep, should be taken. Put sleep first. Don't take the opportunity to dust or tidy the bedroom.

Signs of fatigue or lack of sleep are, for example, that you find you are not enjoying music when you usually like it, or feel too tired to read or go out with your husband to see friends, even if you can take the baby with you. The extra work involved in caring for a baby, the broken nights and the anxiety and mental strain of coping – all conspire to create exhaustion. Even an hour's good sleep during the day helps. It is also important to take physical care of yourself, and make sure you have at least one good meal a day and get out for a short walk.

Care should be taken not to add to physical exhaustion by moving house at this time; or by looking after ill or elderly relatives; or carrying out any unnecessary tasks; or trying to maintain outside activities at pre-birth level and failing to cut down on the number of responsibilities these entail; or failing to arrange in advance for baby-sitting needs; or spending too much time trying to keep up appearances, both in the house and personally. Don't feel guilty at using disposable nappies or convenience foods, as these are useful short cuts.

It gives people pleasure to help mothers with new babies. If, as a new mother, a friend offers to do your nappies for you, or take the new baby or the other toddler for a walk, *accept*. Some mothers, afraid of appearing inadequate and unable to cope, reject help. Consider it as a way of cementing friendship rather than as an implication that you are an incompetent mother. Try to get to know other mothers who are experienced at bringing up children.

Setting time aside for relaxation, to lower anxiety and fear when coping with the baby at home, is important. Relaxation will probably have been practised at antenatal classes and the same methods can be used at home.

There is often a 'last-straw' – a row with a husband, outrageous behaviour by the baby or non-stop crying, bad news of some kind – and the mother may suddenly reach the end of her tether. It is important at this stage to get practical help – from a health visitor, doctor, the local National Childbirth Trust, a neighbour, a mutual-help organisation, a social worker – rather than just hope that the situation will improve. Reducing the amount of work to be done also reduces tension.

There is an obvious risk to the baby in this situation. A mother may have no other way of expressing angry feelings than to take them out on the baby. This then creates even more unacceptable feelings of guilt. Mothers really need to 'talk out' these feelings. Parents Anonymous – a telephone help-line for parents who are at the end of their tether and feel like battering, or have battered, their children – can be of immense help here. Those answering the calls are mothers who have been in exactly the same situation themselves. (*See Appendix II for addresses and details.*)

Some mothers will rely on tranquillisers at this stage but, although these reduce tension, they can also have the effect of releasing inhibitions. 'I felt lovely and floaty after taking tranquillisers,' one young mother told me, 'and I came home and nearly tossed my baby out of the window.'

Sometimes a mother will confide in the doctor at her family planning or health clinic. Health visitors often notice when a mother starts coming into the clinic more often than is strictly necessary, recognising this as a sign that the mother needs to talk to someone. A mother may avoid asking a health visitor to call, not wishing to admit to her state of mind. But health visitors are trained to notice when things are going awry.

One London-based health visitor said: 'Very often they are not caring for themselves, have a general air of not coping, are not organised and are often very fearful, especially when the baby is new. This kind of mother is constantly on the phone to you because the baby won't take as much milk as she thinks it should. And things have tended to pile up. This is where our home visiting is so useful. It's easier for them to talk there and it shows you are interested. And while you are talking, you can help with the washing up, or folding nappies. That kind of practical help is really needed. Sometimes you'll chat for an hour and, just as you're about to leave, they'll blurt out about their depression.'

As well as practical advice and information, new mothers need encouragement and approval – from husbands, friends, neighbours and relations. Anyone doing a new job lacks confidence. Actors, on first nights, need flattering about their performance to be able to face the second night. The same kind of positive support is essential for mothers who feel frightened and believe they are coping inadequately (a major cause of depression).

One way of getting this support, if it does not come from friends or relations, is to join a women's group or a mother-and-toddler group, or contact the nearest National Childbirth Trust group. It is a way of getting practical tips and, if not of solving worries, at least of sharing them. The need for such outlets is evident in the fast growth of the relatively new organisation called Mama.

If nothing like this exists in your area, and you feel in need of more formal help, ask your doctor where the nearest group therapy is available and if he will refer you; or contact a counsellor (through the British Association of Counsellors).

There is nothing to be ashamed of in post-natal depression. The nearest young mother down the street is probably concealing the fact that she feels exactly the same way. The important point is not to cover it up, but to get help.

7

Anorexia

One of the first descriptions of anorexia nervosa was by a seventeenth-century physician, who called it a 'nervous consumption' caused by 'sad and anxious cares'. Anorexia nervosa (anorexia is from the Greek, meaning 'lack of appetite') is a condition in which there is a profound aversion to food, often leading to severe self-starvation and emaciation. Sufferers will rigidly control the amount they eat, and have an abnormal fear of regaining normal weight. As one schoolgirl said, 'I would eat a little breakfast and then nothing for the rest of the day. My starvation was so intense, I could hardly think.'

AGE AT ONSET

Anorexia nervosa rarely begins before the start of puberty (which is between nine and thirteen for most girls). Usually the onset is after menstruation and body changes, like breast development, have taken place. Studies of schoolgirls show that about one in every 200 is anorexic, frequently in the 16–18 age group. Many girls in their early twenties also suffer from the condition, but it is comparatively rare after that. Nevertheless, there are known cases of women in their fifties and sixties who are anorexic. It is not confined to those – of whatever age – who have not had sexual experience. Of new cases admitted to one Bristol clinic, some 10 per cent were married women, who had only become anorexic after marriage (and, in two-fifths of the cases, after having had one or more children); one was an unmarried mother; and two were practising homosexuals (one male, one female).

SEX RATIO

Both males and females suffer from anorexia, but it is estimated that only some 7 per cent of anorexics are males. One reason for this may be that if the cause of anorexia is linked to the acceptance of an adult role, with a fear of sexual maturity (*see* Causes, *below*), men do not have to face the trauma of breast development, menstruation, pregnancy, giving birth and breast-feeding. Studies also show, however, that three times more men than women reveal no change in appetite when under stress.

EFFECTS

Physical effects include drastic weight loss, hyperactivity, amenorrhoea (cessation of menstruation), constipation, dizziness (caused by lack of food), dehydration (lack of food and fluid), oedema (swelling of tissues with fluid, particularly noticeable on face, ankles and stomach, due to lack of protein). In extreme cases, hair and teeth can fall out and a light growth of downy hair can appear on the back of hands and forearms. Cuts and bruises can take weeks to disappear or heal. Anorexia is an extremely serious condition and can, unchecked, result in death.

Anorexia also has an effect mentally. The mind becomes disturbed and logic is impaired. Anorexics, even when emaciated, are still intent on losing weight and, even if they look at themselves in the mirror, cannot see themselves as thin. Their view of themselves is at variance with reality.

CAUSES

DEPENDENCY

There is no single, or agreed, cause of anorexia. But traditionally one of the fundamental psychological factors is the refusal to grow up. By not eating, it is argued, the girl has found a way to remain a girl by shedding her curves and her periods. But, as one doctor who counsels anorexics says: 'I find it impossible to say that the girl restricts her eating with the purpose of losing her periods when she does not know at the time she starts to cut down on eating that there is any connection between the two.'

It is perhaps clearer to explain this element of anorexia as being the difficulty of leaving the role of the dependent child and entering adulthood, of having to think and act independently and responsibly. Anorexia, for instance, is particularly prevalent among offspring of overprotective parents. It can also set in when a person becomes a parent, with the attendant responsibilities; or when a middle-aged person loses a parent, and has to 'grow up'. Many parents of children with anorexia have difficulty in allowing them to grow up, referring to them as 'our child' when they are in their mid-twenties or even their forties.

PERSONALITY CHARACTERISTICS

What is it that turns a person towards anorexia, rather than some other kind of breakdown or rebellion? A contributory cause is character and emotional make-up. Anorexics are, above all, perfectionists. They need to do something well and set themselves impossible goals. Yet even when they get high marks at school or university they consider them not high enough; and if someone compliments them on their looks they disregard the remark, feeling they are not attractive enough. They think they could do better: they regard themselves with disgust as failures. They have no self-esteem or self-confidence. And as, fundamentally, they do not like themselves, they do not see that others can. Even when offered friendship, they consider that this is because people 'feel sorry for them'. They dislike displays of feeling and value remaining in control. By losing weight, they think they can become more attractive; can prove their will-power; and can show they are effectively in control.

WORK PRESSURES

The anorexic's need to do well is usually in response to the parents' high expectations of their attainments, both socially and academically. Academically, the really serious pressure begins in the teens, when examination success and future career are constant topics of conversation. Stress (resulting in loss of appetite), guilt (because of not doing even better in exams) and the need to impose control on an existence which shows sudden, alarming signs of getting out of control lead to the need to control some other aspect of their life, such as their physical form.

One girl of twenty, for example, said that she was terrified of failing exams at university and had become very depressed. She became hyperactive, studying at night and going for long walks during the day, and she practically stopped eating. 'I just floated around, looking thin and missing lectures.' Only after she opted out of university did her weight stabilise. She then managed to get a good job but, though successful at it, she 'felt something was going to happen. It was going too well and I was afraid of it going out of control. And the thing you control most is your weight, so I kept it down to show I *could* keep things in control.'

Another girl, who had suffered from anorexia but had managed to keep her weight at a certain reasonable (to her) level, then came under more pressure at work. Writing in the Anorexic Aid newsletter, she said: 'I had changed my job and felt that I was not coping with the new one very well and at the back of my mind I knew if I became anorexic again I could not be blamed for any mistakes I made, as I was ill.'

FIGURE CONSCIOUSNESS

Being overweight is an unacceptable condition for many girls who lack self-confidence and self-esteem. Such girls are very figure-conscious and feel that if only they could be slim – or slimmer – they would be as attractive as they feel other people are. Attractiveness equals slimness in their minds, reinforced by the media's preoccupation with the slim beauty. Being fat, in Western culture, is not considered attractive, as it is in other cultures where there is less to eat.

One girl described her attitude this way: 'I had a firm conviction that fat was ugly, ludicrous, and disabling. And thin was wonderful. My mother's attempts to reconcile me to obesity – she would flourish Rubens and Renoir nudes before me and read aloud enticing descriptions of fat women from Victorian novels – I regarded with extreme suspicion. . . . Nevertheless, since enough is enough, she got me a proper diet sheet from a doctor and, with encouragement from my family, I embarked on a disastrous course.'

Her weight fell from fifteen stone to five and a half in nine months. 'I had set out on this crazy species of self-mortification out of pure sexual vanity. Consciously, at least . . . I assumed that no man in his right mind could ever have been attracted to Fat Angie; therefore I reduced myself to a physical condition – that of Walking Corpse – that only a chronic necrophile could have fancied.'

Another girl said that in her case it had all started when she was about sixteen: 'I was a well-built girl and my mother said it was just puppy fat and I would grow out of it. But all my friends were talking about boys and I wanted to be "in" as well. Until then I had been preoccupied with school. Then I read an article in a women's magazine about dieting – just eating protein and nothing else. I tried it secretly – putting the vegetables and spuds into a paper tissue and just eating the meat, and so on – and that's how it started.'

Many insecure young girls go to discos or youth clubs wearing attractive clothes to give themselves confidence. If they are still lacking partners, they decide it is due to their figure. They start losing weight, still feel unattractive, so lose some more. But they never seem to attain the 'right' weight to build up their confidence: when they are seven stone, they want to be six stone thirteen. And so it goes on. One girl explained it this way: 'I remember as a child envying another school-friend and thinking, "I want to be like her." I felt an absolute nothing. I had no self-esteem. I used to watch the girls on the beaches: they were so attractive and thin.'

Non-existent or fragile self-confidence naturally makes girls particularly vulnerable to a passing comment about their looks or figure. One girl, whose weight at one point went down to around four stone, recalled being touchy about food in her late teens, but said that it was a chance remark by her boyfriend that set her off dieting. 'He happened to say one day, "You're the right weight now, but don't for goodness sake put on any more." And I was lacking in confidence and decided to go on a diet, because then I felt he would be even more pleased with me. And there was a banana diet in one of those women's magazines and I stuck to this and I thought, this is easy. And at lunch time I was having half a banana and another half for dinner and lots of coffee and all the time my weight was going down and down and I was feeling very depressed.'

Another teenager said that it hadn't occurred to her to diet until her boyfriend made comments about her weight: 'I wasn't noticeably overweight, but he was always raving over girls with skinny figures, making me feel grotesque.' One girl in her late teens, noticeably large, became progressively upset 'because there was a lot of talk in the office about my being overweight. Our boss used to call me, "Big Liz". I decided to go on a diet to lose enough weight to buy all the nice clothes the rest of the girls were wearing.'

With those predisposed towards anorexia, starting to diet is the trigger point. One seventeen-year-old who started to follow a diet said: 'I was very strict with myself: only one small meal a day without potatoes or pudding, and absolutely no sweets at any time. I was down to six stone from eight and a half within eight months and my friends and family warned me about the risk of anorexia. But by this time I had become quite obsessive about starving myself to a stupid extreme and had a mental block against eating. All the time I wanted to lose just a little more.'

One other way that sufferers will try to lose weight is to use up as much energy as possible. One girl even refused to use an electric typewriter at work because she thought a manual one would use up more of her energy. Another would leave for work in the morning very early and then get out of the bus after a few stops and walk the rest of the way.

SECRECY AND SOCIAL ISOLATION

Such girls have a need to keep their actions secret, fearing, somehow, that their control over their eating could be wrested from them if found out. Their life turns into one of lies and evasion. They are constantly claiming they have eaten when they have not, or that they do not feel hungry; or giving precise, almost loving details of meals they have not eaten. This naturally leads to social isolation, because most meetings with friends involve meals or at least a cup of tea or coffee. Some girls go out to meals with boyfriends, disappear afterwards in order to make themselves vomit, and might keep up this behaviour for months without revealing the truth. But such girls, with their own strong feelings of self-hatred, find friendship and relationships hard to maintain.

RELATIONSHIP DIFFICULTIES

The obedient, well behaved child of overprotective parents is particularly vulnerable. A docile acceptance of parental authority is often behind the child's wish to assert some sort of control over her life – and the easiest, if not the only, thing to control is appetite. Many have a forceful personality, which is just suppressed. One schoolgirl, whose hair had come out in handfuls and whose teeth became loose after her weight dropped from ten stone eleven to six stone ten, was the daughter of very protective parents, whom she was eager to please. Only after leaving home for university did her weight stabilise. She said: 'I'm beginning now to accept and like myself for the first time, as after two years away from home I realise I am acceptable to other people and not just family.'

Other emotional problems at home can also provoke the need to be in control. One girl, whose father's constant criticism had totally undermined her confidence, lost several stone in weight. Moving away from home to a flat was a considerable help, so was establishing a good relation with a boyfriend; but when this fell through her weight dropped again. A teenager whose weight had dropped to below six stone but who was gradually improving found that she still 'used' anorexia: 'If I have a row with my parents, I just put down my plate.'

Another girl had been extremely upset by her mother's death, particularly as her father seemed to have little time or interest in her, and her weight began to fall. 'I became preoccupied with my weight and would feel desperate if I put on even one pound. I'd weigh myself a few times every week just to make sure. When I was on my diet, I seldom thought of my mother and I would say to myself, "Well at long last I am getting over her not being around." But I knew that if she had been alive she would have noticed how thin I was getting and known something was wrong.' Her feelings were endorsed by a 21-year-old girl who said that after her mother had died two years previously 'my eating just got worse and worse and now all I eat is sometimes mashed potato or a small dish of custard'.

Acting virtually as a marriage counsellor to her parents, who were unhappily married, compounded by problems at school and with her boyfriend, caused one seventeen-year-old's weight to veer erratically. She lost two and a half stone initially then when her parents decided to divorce, 'started eating all the food I had previously forbidden myself'.

BINGEING AND PURGING

Once someone's iron control breaks in a reaction against semi-starvation, she can eat uncontrollably. And usually she eats the very things she has been at most pains to avoid: food which is rich with protein or starch. One girl who kept to an almost starvation diet during the week would visit her mother at weekends and eat vast quantities of whatever she could find in her cupboards and fridge – admitting that after the binge she absolutely loathed herself Another wrote down in despair: 'Today, 12.30 p.m. in my lunch break, I ate one Cadbury Flake, one Picnic, one Kit Kat, one cheese and pickle roll, one sausage roll, one doughnut, one Topic, one fruit yogurt, one piece of cheesecake, one packet of crisps, one Bounty, one bag of McDonalds french fries, two Coca-Colas, one more packet of crisps. I then made myself vomit. Why do I do it?'

The reason that this girl and others purge themselves by laxatives or make themselves vomit after such a binge is to wipe the binge out – to get back in control of their eating and their weight. Their immense feelings of guilt at going on a binge cause them to punish themselves still further by going on an even stricter diet, which leads in turn to another binge. One woman, who started to binge after the birth of her child, said: 'It is like living in a nightmare. When I am on a binge, I can start with an orange and then eat everything in sight. Then I feel even more guilty and depressed and make myself sick by drinking vinegar and soapy water.'

Another anorexic made sure that she always started her binges by eating red carrots or red pickled cabbage. Only when she had brought everything up – including, finally, the red carrots or cabbage with which she knew she had begun – did she feel purged of her action. Once this vicious circle of starving – bingeing – purging starts, it seems unstoppable. 'When I get into stuffing then vomiting, for days non-stop, except to sleep, I fear for my life,' said one woman.

What is particularly frightening to those concerned is that, in a life devoted to rigid control of eating, they are suddenly overwhelmed by an *uncontrollable* need to eat. They are terrified that, once they start to eat, they will genuinely be unable to stop: it is similar to the alcoholic's fear of the result of taking one drink. This uncontrollability can spread to other areas of their lives. Sufferers at this stage often lose control of their spending and run up overdrafts or loans for no real reason. They might, in extreme cases, even steal food from super-markets – though this adds to their strong feelings of self-disgust and shame.

COMPULSIVE EATING

The pressures that cause self-starvation can also cause compulsive eating – though this is not necessarily attended by bingeing. One overweight nineteen-year-old, for example, ate so obsessively when she went to university that she gave up the degree course. She finally returned to a polytechnic to study, but said that she was 'so gripped by my problem that instead of staying with my college friends at weekends and going out in the evenings I go to my family home so I can stay in and eat. I do not even enjoy eating any more, but just eat and eat everything in sight. I am extremely shy with most people and worry an awful lot – though I don't know if I am shy because I find myself totally unattractive, or if my shyness causes my overeating.'

A younger girl, who said that she had left school 'after realising I could never sort out all the schoolwork I had not done', started to eat compulsively to overcome her depression. An unhappy home life, with constantly quarrelling parents, worsened matters. 'For several months, I was stealing piles and piles of food, and was eventually taken to court.' However, since she started working, she has slowly settled down and has started to relate to other people and make friends.

An eighteen-year-old, the only child of devoted parents, found she could not cope at university and left to take a secretarial job, which she despised. She felt that she had failed her parents and, always rather overweight, began to eat compulsively. Treatment was feared because she thought her parents 'would cringe at the thought of my being mentally unstable'. She eats compulsively, she says, because 'firstly, I feel warm and safe; secondly, it will not let me down; thirdly, I feel drowsy and can forget reality; fourthly, habit'.

Another girl, who also needed food for comfort, to compensate for an unhappy home background, said: 'In the mornings, I used to feel terrible from eating so much the previous day; but this would not stop me from eating every bit as much, and even more, the next day. I'd buy large cakes and eat them all in my room and dozens of buns and bread and butter.'

Eating like this *is* a comfort, a way of giving oneself a private treat to make up for the unkindness of life. Violet creams, chocolate sauce, iced cakes – a sugar-plum fairy-cake land. Only when the person takes steps to change the unhappy situation which is behind the need for comfort will the need to eat compulsively end.

TREATMENT FOR ANOREXIA

Sufferers can be successfully treated only when they themselves seek help. This might be when they have reached a very low weight and feel so weak and so lacking in energy that they cannot face going on like this; or it may be that they finally realise the dangerous situation they are in. Sometimes, their fear of their uncontrollable eating needs frightens them into asking for treatment.

Without their co-operation, however, long-term success is unlikely. First, they conceal the early and middle stages, when the condition is more susceptible to treatment ('I am too ashamed to discuss it with friends'; 'I cannot tell the doctor about this'; 'I couldn't possibly tell my husband or family about this as I know they would be really mad'). Second, if sent to hospital against their wishes, their attitude remains that they are not ill. As one girl said: 'When I walked into hospital, I couldn't understand what people were talking about: four stone three was large as far as I was concerned. I was more intent on getting it down than thinking I was on the danger level. Admitting it was to admit that I was out of control, and control was the keyword for me. I had to control the point on the scales.'

However, when someone is at danger level with her weight, the first step has to be to get her to hospital to save her life and raise her weight to a more normal level. This is usually done by putting her on standard – even double – portions of food. However, this can be very frightening ('though in one way, I was very relieved', said one girl, who had been in a special anorexic unit, 'because I had to eat, it wasn't my fault, I couldn't blame myself').

The other advantages of hospital are that the person is taken away from the situation which has caused the disorder; and at some hospitals psychotherapy and counselling services are available. Without the help of a therapist, sufferers will retain their obsessional attitude towards food, and regress once home. Indeed, they are quite intelligent and manipulative enough to beat the system while still in hospital. One girl said: 'You'd be taught by the others in the unit what to say to the consultants so that you could get out. They would say, "How do you feel about your weight?" and I would say, "I realise it must go up." Positive thinking, that's what they wanted. And the dieticians would say, "What can you eat?" and you'd ask for soft-boiled eggs. That way you could pierce the shell and let the yellow go into the egg cup and eat the white, which hadn't any calories.'

If the therapeutic help received in hospital is not successful, the sufferer will regress on return home. One girl, whose weight had gone up three stone before she was allowed to leave hospital, said she hated herself when she left: 'My stomach was bloated and I felt a freak.' She returned to her old habits on being faced with her first meal at home. 'My mother had made an effort, and gave me soup and a little chicken. I remember trying to hide the chicken under the skin and avoiding the peas in the soup.'

The realisation that her future life could mean incessant trips to hospital made her take an overdose of the antidepressants given to her by the hospital. Taken back there, this time she saw a psychologist, 'who was interested in me and not just my weight'. He made it clear to her that she had to start learning to get out of the hospital and think of the future, and herself as an individual. As the girl herself admitted, 'I had never lost my temper as a child and during this period I was going through a lot of childhood and adolescent feelings. I had found it hard to face maturity.'

The psychologist visited her parents and, when she felt able to leave the hospital, suggested she stayed with a cousin, considering it bad for her to return to the same situation at home. She was still barely seven stone, and counted calories obsessively as she believed the psychologist would reject her if she put on too much weight. It took over a year before her weight and confidence reached a normal level. Both weight gain and counselling were very gradual, without there being too much of one or the other, to enable a stable recovery to take place.

In treating this girl, the psychologist in question put the emphasis on five main points. First, individuality. He concentrated on the problems that were unique to her. Second, motivation. If the anorexic was dissatisfied with her present behaviour, she must want to change it before this can be accomplished. Third, dependency. He had to be prepared to take on the total dependency of the patient. Fourth, he had to give the patient a belief in her own capacity to change and the likely success of that change. Fifth, he had to encourage the patient to become independent.

A social worker, in talking about those with anorexia on her case list, said: 'The quality of their life is very grey and very limited; and the only thing I feel I can do is give them some dignity and increase their interest in life. Some of the younger ones, who have not yet become chronic anorexics, I can help just by talking to them, by giving them a lot of time, and allowing them to put on weight very, very slowly.'

There is still need for counselling or therapy, by individuals or groups, after discharge from hospital. One such group was set up by Eileen Vaughan, a part-time counsellor at a polytechnic, to look at the emotional difficulties underlying anorexia. She describes the outcome in her article, 'Counselling Anorexia'. Her first group included some parents as well as anorexics, but was not really successful owing to the – often unacknowledged – hostility between them (though very few of those in the group were able to face up to admitting malaise in the family). Mothers tended to answer for their daughters, who seemed lacking in independence. (One mother still bathed her seventeen-year-old daughter and washed her hair; another provided meals for her married children – two of whom had anorexia.) Parents were angry at the waste of their daughters' lives – making the daughters angry, in turn, at believing they were valued for their achievements and not themselves. Group members needed reassurance from one another. This was also required in a second group – this time of anorexic girls alone – where a strong picture emerged of very low self-image and despair.

Anorexics, bewildered, frightened, or even disgusted by their own behaviour, also need reassurance that their behaviour is not unique; and they can find it through the Anorexic Aid organisation, which holds group meetings in towns throughout the country. 'Everyone who goes to Anorexic Aid meetings has been through it,' said one of the organisers. 'We're not trying to force anyone attending to eat, but just give them a chance to talk to others who have got better and discuss their problems with them, if they feel like it. I was amazed myself, when I first went to a meeting, to find others like myself. It was such a relief.'

A close friend, who has the trust of the person with anorexia, can sometimes help her to recover. In one such case, a working colleague, who knew the wife was deceiving her husband about the amount she was eating, tried to get her to see the doctor. When this failed, she persuaded the woman – who was frightened and anxious to co-operate – to agree to eat a little toast and coffee for breakfast, and small portions of meat and two vegetables for lunch and dinner. She also promised to weigh herself only once a day, relaying this information to the colleague; and also to telephone her to talk about her feelings whenever she faced the need to overeat, or cut down further, and to call in one evening a week to talk. Sufferers usually require more deep-rooted counselling than this, but such help would at least provide reassurance and move them out of the eating habit groove they are in.

PRACTICAL POINTS

A person with anorexia can be so devious that parents or friends may be unaware of what is happening until weight loss has become drastic. But pointers that something is wrong are:

1 Is the person at the table at meal times, or has she argued or made an excuse not to eat with the family? (For example, she may say that she has eaten a lot at lunch that day, met a friend and had supper out; still feels full from a restaurant lunch, is not really hungry at the moment; she will ask if she *must* always eat with you, say she will make something for herself later, doesn't really like the food you serve up, is really very well and likes being thin.)

2 Is she constantly reading slimming magazines, trying out diets?

3 Is she spending a lot of time in health shops, or insisting on low calorie food and drinks? Does she avoid bread and potatoes and keep on a strict regime?

4 Is she vomiting after meals, or disappearing to a lavatory even in a restaurant?

TO CUT DOWN LIKELIHOOD OF ANOREXIA

1 Do not make your children feel guilty about any sacrifices you may have made for them.

2 Avoid pressurising them to do well, socially or academically.

3 Do not be over-protective and encourage dependency.

IF ANOREXIA HAS SET IN

Because those concerned do not regard weight loss as a problem, they

1   will only deny it if challenged. If they are drastically thin, they may need to go to hospital to have their life saved. It may be wise to talk the matter over with a therapist or Anorexic Aid to discover what stage they are at.

2   Only people the sufferers trust and like will be able to help – and they will need to emphasise that they are not trying to interfere, to force the sufferer to eat, but that they just want to help. (It is useless, for instance, commenting on the habit of playing with food at the table; it is better to ignore this rather than use pressure.)

3   The sufferer needs to be encouraged to see a therapist or counsellor, or go to an Anorexic Aid group; but if the relation or friend does it all, the sufferer will not bother to carry it through. It is best to offer a leaflet, or the address of a therapist, and just suggest, when he or she feels able, contacting that address for help.

4   Information about the condition, as well as information on local groups, can be obtained from the headquarters of Anorexic Aid.

5   The Women's Therapy Centre, in London, organises self-help groups on the theme of compulsive eating.

6   The important, positive point for parents – and ultimately the anorexic – to realise is that it is possible to reverse the process and be cured.

8

The Elderly Mentally Infirm

The problems of mental ill-health among the elderly are too frequently dismissed with: 'Well, what can you expect at that age?' Depression, for example, is described as being 'natural'. Doctors tend to explain it by saying that the body is run down, depression is only to be expected, and write it off as due to old age.

But the attitude that mental ill-health is inevitably linked with old age has led to a less positive approach in treating the elderly. Most forms of mental disability *can* be helped by treatment. Yet elderly people will often not admit their problems, as they themselves regard these as 'insoluble'. In a study carried out by Peter Townsend and Dorothy Wedderburn in 1962, it was found that elderly people frequently underestimated the seriousness of their condition, or deliberately refrained from asking advice in case this led to a greater dependence on others. And a Scottish study of the elderly, in 1964, found that general practitioners knew nothing about 60 per cent of the neuroses, 76 per cent of the depressions and 87 per cent of dementias, which were present among their elderly patients.

CONFUSION

Confusion in the elderly, like depression, is also often written off as something to be expected. In psychiatric terms, confusion means actual disorientation. If someone is slightly vague or slow, or has poor concentration or memory, that is not classified as confusion.

An acute state of confusion should always be referred to a doctor. This is especially so if periods of confusion alternate with lucid intervals, because the condition is potentially curable. Such confusion frequently has a physical cause – for example, anaemia, pneumonia, bruising, a broken bone, heart trouble, kidney disease, taking too little fluid, infection, or the side-effects of drugs. It is up to the doctor to trace the cause. One woman, for example, went into a state of confusion prior to a diabetic coma. Once it was realised that diabetes was behind the confusion, the woman was transferred to accommodation where special diabetic meals were prepared. Because those involved – whether social workers, doctors or relatives – sometimes do not have enough patience to take down the history which has led to the confusion, old people are often dismissed as senile. There is the feeling that there is no need to investigate.

Elderly people who are less acutely confused, but are vague and muddled because of poor memory and the anxieties this brings, need careful watching if living on their own, because they could obviously cause themselves harm: the gas can be left on, a lighted candle left on, the bath allowed to overflow, or cigarettes left to burn. In these circumstances, if the person concerned is living on his own, he needs to be admitted to some kind of care.

DEPRESSION

Depression is the most common mental disorder affecting people between sixty-five and seventy-five. What it is important to stress, however, is that depressive illness in old age is just as amenable to treatment as when it occurs in young people. But all too often depression in the elderly is overlooked. It may be regarded as just merely a normal condition of old age. Symptoms can range from feelings of anxiety, hopelessness, and lack of confidence on one hand, through to delusions and thoughts of suicide. Dr Richard Hunter, writing in *Modern Geriatrics*, says: 'Patients, too, overwork the term depression and it is essential to enquire exactly how and where the patient feels "depressed". It is surprising how often they point to their stomach or chest and one can go on from there. Often it merely means a general malaise, the causes of which may lie in the patient or in his environment.'

Depression even in young people leads to poor concentration, indecisiveness and poor memory. So naturally, when these symptoms occur in an older person where, to a certain extent, they are present already through natural ageing processes, they may suggest more dementia (*see below*) than is actually present.

Richard Hunter points out that in diagnosis 'It is important not to mistake apathy for depression. The term depression is almost too readily bandied about. Often it describes not what the doctor sees, but how he interprets what he sees. . . . Little things which the patient would previously have taken in his stride may begin to worry him and he may find it difficult to shift his mind off them. Such a patient may retail a long catalogue of woes and the mental picture may be dominated by anxiety and depression. Behind it, however, lies the fact that he is not what he used to be, and the cause of this requires investigation because it may be treatable or at least it will be possible to advise how he may be safeguarded from concerns that are proving too much.'

Some of the symptoms of depression will require medical treatment – constipation, lack of appetite, insomnia and loss of weight, together with various rheumatic aches and pains. And depression can also cause changes in behaviour: an elderly person might become isolated, withdrawn or even hostile. As Leon Epstein says, in *Depression in the Elderly*, 'The picture may be one of apathy, inertia, withdrawal into solitude, and a quiet self-depreciation. The patient's apathetic manner, emotional unresponsiveness, and reluctance to talk or to reply to questions are often attributed to old age rather than depressive illness . . . if the old person has some longstanding personality problems and has always shown a tendency to react to disappointments and difficulties by feeling depressed, a depression in old age may be regarded as just one more instance in a familiar pattern. In either case, the treatable aspect of the depression is likely to be overlooked.'

Loss is the main reason for depression in old age. And the most important of these losses is naturally bereavement, as this leaves the remaining spouse without companionship. The deaths of old friends can also be very upsetting, and indeed so can the 'loss' that takes place at retirement when contacts with colleagues come to an end. A feeling of social isolation can set in if there are fewer visits from friends or relatives, because of travel costs among other reasons. 'All I want to do is die,' said one 78-year-old woman. 'My children haven't visited me for weeks; after all I've done for them, they don't care.' A lack of mobility also prevents the more elderly themselves from getting around. Poor eyesight and poor hearing add to the feeling of being cut off. Stress causes depression too – the stress of poor housing conditions, for example, or anxiety about death. And, sometimes, indeed, there is reason enough for unhappiness. One elderly woman told me that she had lost both her husband and best woman friend within the last year; her son had had a serious car accident and had to walk on crutches; and she herself had become too arthritic to cope, and had just been admitted to a geriatric ward in hospital. Her will to live had obviously – and understandably – gone.

A. Goldfarb, in *Geriatric Psychiatry*, finds that most elderly depressed patients get considerable temporary, and in some cases lasting, benefit from appropriate antidepressive treatment. Certainly, antidepressants, tranquillisers and sedatives can produce dramatic results. But in elderly people the destruction of drugs by the body slows down, so a build-up of drugs can take place. Many old people are prescribed certain drugs certain numbers of times a day, and it is easy for them, if living on their own, to get muddled about the dosage and take far too many. Ask the doctor if the person can take his antidepressants at night, to allow a good sleep.

Side-effects of drugs also tend to be magnified in the elderly. One woman of seventy-three, for example, was being treated by her doctor for Parkinson's disease. Finding her confused, and subject to occasional delusions, her doctor called in a hospital geriatrician – who found that the so-called Parkinson's disease, for which she was taking pills, was a side-effect of previously prescribed antidepressants.

Electroconvulsive treatment can be successful with elderly people, but it may impair the memory more than it does with younger people.

Certain symptoms of depression such as weight loss or pains require medical treatment. For instance, if the patient complains of a headache which is coupled with depression, this could be caused by a tumour. Or, if a personality change is accompanied by disturbed behaviour, it could be a late onset of epilepsy (even without fits). Agitated depression could be due to developing diabetes, or vitamin-B deficiency.

However, medical treatment on its own may be insufficient. It is also necessary to alleviate social isolation by alerting social workers – who can help with both practical and emotional problems, and organise a home help – and voluntary organisations. These organisations can be immensely useful – running Darby and Joan Clubs, visiting the elderly, organising meals on wheels. Going to a day centre can also help prevent a feeling of isolation.

DEMENTIA AND AGEING

Dementia is a frightening word. As T. G. Judge pointed out in *Drugs and Dementia*, 'Originally it was used to mean "loss of mind" but it has come to mean "irreversible loss of mind" and unfortunately many people regard it as a final diagnostic label indicating that neither further investigation is required nor is treatment possible.'

There are two main reasons for dementia. First, the arteries of the brain can become diseased and fail to provide the brain with enough blood (arteriosclerotic dementia). Second, there can be a degenerative process in the brain (senile dementia). The brain grows smaller, ages, and the cells that die cannot be replaced.

Dementia of either variety affects more than one person in five of those aged over eighty. A gradual deterioration in performance, however, is likely to have begun from the sixties. This is due to ageing or 'senescence'. Dr Carrick McDonald, who is the area psycho-geriatrician for Croydon, believes that dementia is this same process of ageing, but telescoped into five or six years rather than ten or twenty. The normal pattern of deterioration usually progresses through the following stages:

1 Memory disturbance.
2 Lack of flexibility of attitudes or reasoning power. People will do things the way they always did them, even if inappropriate. For

example, a man who was a councillor might behave as if he still was one. There is a repetition of behaviour which has been successful in the past, though it is not any longer. This appears to others as obstinacy or rigidity.

3   Not being able to find the right words. For instance, describing a watch as 'This is for telling the time'. General language difficulties.

4   Loss of skills. For example, people will start to dress in-appropriately, perhaps putting pants on over frocks, or are unable to get into a jacket.

5   Loss of control over bladder and bowels.

6   The last thing to go is elementary social responses, like rising when expected to rise, or turning away when you are coughing.

In Dr McDonald's own experience, 50 per cent of the people he is called to see suffer from senescence; 40 per cent from dementia and the remaining 10 per cent from other states such as confusion or depression.

There is a grey area between senescence and dementia. 'But if senile dementia is diagnosed,' says Dr McDonald, 'I expect the person to go downhill rapidly. So I expect to admit these people into hospital because I don't believe any domestic situation can stand the strain of double incontinence. I make sure I tell relations the facts: my guess as to when the person may die. People feel guilty at putting relations into hospital, so they get angry with the staff and create all sorts of problems. They feel, "What have I done to Mum?" I tell them that the elderly person concerned is going to go downhill. When they ask if anything can be done, I say no; go anywhere and it will happen. I explain that there will be no pain. I think it's a good way to go, even though it's upsetting to watch.

'In deciding whether or not an elderly person should go to hospital, you have to balance the patient's danger to themselves – for example, are they likely to fall downstairs? – with the effect hospital may have on them. But if you decide their own surroundings are still important, then I believe the patient should have the dignity of running that risk. An angry daughter may disagree: she may not be able to tolerate the idea of her mother falling down. But as soon as you change the surroundings, the patient will go very quickly down for a spell. You take them away from all the things that orientate them to their past life.'

Very often, dementia causes a crisis. A family may suddenly decide that the limit of their tolerance has been reached; the main caring relative may have become ill; a patient living alone may have been discharged from hospital and be unable to cope on her own; the elderly person may have had a stroke or some other illness; or there may not have been enough help forthcoming from local services.

A doctor is usually informed by a relative, or neighbour, when dementia gets to a serious state – and the patient, or relatives, can no longer manage. On a house call by a geriatrician that I attended myself, the assessment of the patient – a woman of seventy five – was quite detailed. A short physical examination took place – blood pressure was taken and reflexes measured. The patient was a small, rather nervous woman, whom the doctor had reported as being in need of assessment because she was confused about her sister's recent death, had fallen once in the surgery, and had a previous history of depression. When questioned about her sister, she explained that she was lonely and still 'talked' to her sister for companionship. The geriatrician asked to see all the pills she was taking and found she had a store of different ones, including tranquillisers and antidepressants. Taken together, as she was doing, these may well have led to some of her confusion.

The geriatrician then carried out a brief 'mental check', asking for example, if she could remember the design on the newly issued Christmas stamp (she was writing her Christmas cards at the time); and if she could take seven from a hundred, and then another seven from the figure she gave. He next tactfully checked out how much food she had in the larder. Tom Arie mentions this point in *Dementia in the Elderly: diagnosis and assessment:* 'If the old person lives alone, the state of her home will often be the best measure of her capacity for self-care (though one must take care to establish what help she is having from others). The kitchen and the contents of the larder are particularly eloquent – what was the last meal, how much of it has been eaten, is there any accumulation of bottles? More generally, is the place clean, is it warm, is there gross neglect of hygiene, signs that the bed had been slept in?'

On the subject of a mental examination, Tom Arie goes on to say: 'The examination must be unhurried and the patient will need a few moments to take in what is happening. . . . A strange man suddenly appearing off the street and immediately asking "What is the name of the Prime Minister?" is likely either to put the final touch to the patient's confusion, or to convince her that she has fallen into the hands of a madman. One should explain carefully who one is. I usually also ask the patient to remember my name, which I then repeat to her, explaining that I will ask her to repeat it for me later, "because I want to see how good your memory is".'

The questions put to elderly people to check on intellectual impairment usually include memory tests (asking their address, then asking for it again ten minutes later); vocabulary test (define the meaning of 'ship', 'remorse'); calculation (subtract 35p from 76p); speech (naming objects on a tray, obeying simple commands); and practical tests (copying patterns with matchsticks).

The way dementia develops varies from person to person. It might show itself in unobtrusive loss of memory and skills, or in more positive psychotic symptoms. Sometimes, an elderly mentally infirm person can suffer from feelings of persecution, in the belief that her neighbours are ganging up on her. Or she may have paranoid feelings that she is being watched or followed. Or claim to hear voices discussing her, or nocturnal visitors, whom she may have invented for company.

AGEING

The earlier stages of ageing, of gradual impairment of the senses, are very subtle. You might have to know the person very well to know that they are not functioning so well. But there are certain changes to look out for: restlessness, sleeplessness and getting up in the night are signs that things are going seriously awry. Sleeping patterns become disturbed and the person starts sleeping at the wrong time.

The correct thing to do is to re-establish the correct sleep pattern by making sure the elderly person does not sleep during the day.

MEMORY DEFICIENCIES

In the elderly, memory deficiencies start with the loss of memory of recent events, and then progress back. Added to this is the difficulty in registering information. An elderly person might think, 'Now the doctor told me to take two tablets a day, one in the morning and one in the evening. Have I taken this morning's tablet?', go to the cupboard to take out the pill – and a quarter of an hour later, do the same thing. In this way, old people can poison themselves, especially with heart tablets and water tablets. And tranquillisers can add to any confusion which already exists.

The elderly person may also tend to go shopping and come back with butter and bread but nothing else, or else go to a post office and collect their pension but forget to buy stamps for their letters.

In these circumstances, older people should be given a calendar or diary which they can tick off when they take prescribed pills. They should also be encouraged to draw up a list of what they need before they go out, to assist their memory. In the early days it is a good idea to have very easily picked-up clues: a big calendar, a clock with a simple face and no second hand, a radio with a loud volume, a lavatory with a distinctive door. Memory cues, like a pinned-up card saying 'GLASSES', may prevent them leaving the house without these.

If memory worsens, a person may become forgetful about simple things about the house. He may, when he goes into the bedroom, forget that there is an oil-fire alight in the sitting-room; or put the tap on in the bathroom and forget having done so; or put the joint in the oven and leave it there.

If a relation or anyone else is living in the same house, they should recognise and watch for these happenings. And change a dangerous gas or oil appliance for a safer electrical one. If a person is living on his own, however, and is a potential danger to himself, it is better if he can go to some kind of sheltered housing where meals can be prepared and where there is a warden in overall charge. In this way, he can keep his basic independence, but have someone watching over him and preventing anything dangerous happening.

Should wandering behaviour set in, this can also be dangerous.

Someone might wander away and not be able to find his way back, or return wet and cold. Eventually he does not come back, or is picked up by the police. Old people are particularly likely to get lost if there have been any substantial changes in the neighbourhood – as these are not remembered, even if they are comparatively nearby. If they have been rehoused, this adds to the problem immensely. They may have known the old district well: in another area, they get lost. Similar problems occur if they are rehoused into a different kind of flat. If it has underfloor heating, for example, with various knobs to turn, they may get frightened of the gadgets, switch them off and stay in a cold flat.

It is important here to explain any new or different gadgets to elderly people, and to do so several times. The same applies to a new neighbourhood: walk with them as often as possible to the places they are most likely to have to visit, such as the post office or supermarket. As far as wandering is concerned, one practical measure is to fit a lock on the door.

Another sign of ageing is when a person repeats the same thing again and again. If you ask question A, you will get the answer. But if you ask question B, you will get the same answer. When a person gets to that stage, he should be assessed. But although you might suggest to old people that they need to see a doctor, they often will not because of obstinacy – and perhaps fear. And, indeed, the more they need treatment, the more rigid they become.

It is best to arrange a house call by a doctor if the person concerned will not go to the doctor. But as far as general attitudes are concerned, once these have become fixed and rigid, it is useless to try and argue. If an elderly person says, for instance, 'I can't be bothered to read the papers, we used to do it better in my day,' it is pointless to argue. This rigidity is a defence against facing the fact that he cannot succeed in the new world.

What happens then is a gradual 'disengagement'. An elderly man, say, would protect himself from failing in this new world by becoming uninvolved, by stopping going to clubs and the bowling, and eventually stopping his visits to his sons or daughters. The family then feels hurt, thinking their father no longer cares.

Another happening that can cause family strains is when the personality traits that a person had when younger become far more exaggerated. If someone has been obstinate, he gets worse; if authoritarian, he becomes domineering. The inhibition effect located at the front of the brain dies. Nothing can be done about this, but it is as well to understand it and not blame the person concerned, or take it personally.

Ageing people pick up infections very quickly. The reserve strength for every bodily function is down, and the brain is being served poorly by a restricted amount of blood. They may suffer from fainting attacks if the lungs are not working properly, and toxic tissue can lead to confusion in the brain. They become apathetic and tired.

Although any confusion must be reported at once to a doctor, it is also important not to criticise any slowness, as this will simply cause a catastrophic reaction. Stress only makes an old person perform worse and you should therefore try to avoid statements like 'You must be ready in five minutes' or 'Can't you see you've done this wrong again.' If someone has their pyjamas on back to front, or gets the day of the week muddled, this should be corrected gently, or you can generate a feeling of panic.

Unfortunately, it is very difficult, with parents, not to feel and act in an irritated manner. You would not react this way with an elderly neighbour, but it is hard to accept that your parents, to whom you once looked up and from whom you learnt, are now becoming progressively more incapable. Because you are upset, and want to stop it happening, you shout at them, which makes them worse.

Another aspect of ageing which often annoys younger people is constant reminiscing about the past. But naturally, if you cannot retain and register new information, you are only going to be able to recall the old days. What is remembered is often embellished, but it means that elderly people are much happier living with their families, who also remember these events, than with strangers.

It is when certain aspects of the past memory begin to fade that the elderly person starts becoming concerned, because she feels she does not know any longer what is going on, who is alive and who is dead. She gets what is called 'projection panic' when she suddenly finds she cannot think about the future. This is understandably a time when thoughts of suicide are expressed. 'I get so muddled and I think I am going,' said one woman in her late seventies. 'But I want to go with all my faculties.' The suicide rate at that age is very high, and relations need to be alert. Very often, in the week or two prior to the attempt, old people often tell a key person that they are 'thinking of doing something'.

One of the most important ways to encourage old people, and raise their self-esteem, is in your attitude to them. If you privately write them off, and talk down to them as if they were children, they will accept themselves as having left the intelligent, adult world. MIND's report *Mental Health for Elderly People* makes this point when referring to treatment in homes and hospitals: 'You go into most old people's homes and you hear elderly citizens being addressed as "Gran", "love" or by their forenames and nicknames without so much as a by-your-leave. Or go into the back wards of many of our depressingly obsolete Victorian mental hospitals and hear nursing staff telling an elderly, demented patient, "We've been a naughty girl today." A similar point is made by John Agate in his book, *Taking Care of Old People at Home*: 'Do not expect an elderly mentally sick person to be able to do all that he used to do; equally, do not assume that he can do nothing. It is good for the mind to be exercised within its current capabilities.'

The St James's Hospital, Leeds, and the Brighton Clinic, Newcastle, among others, use a technique called 'reality orientation' to keep depressed or confused old people in touch with everyday life. It aims at activating living brain cells by stimulation. The idea was originally American and is now being gradually introduced in some hospitals over here. Age Concern and the Royal School of Nursing are interested: the techniques can be used by nurses and therapists, as well as unqualified volunteers. Essentially, they are a gentle bombardment of questions until some kind of response is elicited. Sessions aimed at increasing perception are held daily and stimulation continues on the wards. If a patient asks for a cup of tea, a comment is made, for instance about tea versus coffee, or the time of day it is, or the weather. The technique has proved very successful: some patients in a state of apathy or inertia have, after a fortnight of sessions with one staff member to two old people, been able to take up different interests or even leave the hospital.

Ageing elderly people need companionship, conversation, newspapers, magazines and books if they are not to feel they are degenerating into vegetables. Being on your own most of the day, without any stimulation, naturally slows down your mental processes and adds to any confusion or depression which might be present, due to this loneliness. But a condescending or 'jollying along' attitude does not help. Elderly people, even if verging on mental infirmity, are quick to spot 'do-goodery' visitors. 'Who does she think she's referring to, when she talks about "you old people", said one woman of seventy-one about a young social worker who had been to see her that day. 'I want to be treated as a normal person, and not be told to "Come along, dear".' Another woman in her eighties said: 'I let the schoolchildren come in and watch my television. They are the only ones I see all day, but it keeps me bright just listening to their chatter.' The importance of visiting elderly neighbours, to save them from lonely apathy, cannot be overemphasised.

An article in the *Daily Mail* headlined 'Is power the elixir of life' made the point that many top politicians live on till their seventies or eighties, functioning exceptionally well despite the stress of their jobs. They are surrounded by people who respect, admire – or possibly hate them. But they at least do not meet condescension; nor are they ignored. The same principle should be applied to the average elderly person.

The family's attitude to the elderly parent or relation is of prime importance. Dr Carrick McDonald says that he is called in not only because of the severity of the patient's condition; the tolerance and expectations of relations (and neighbours) also play a part. Some families will tolerate quite bad behaviour. Some will accept a degree of reason, others will not. 'Sometimes it's up to me to judge whether the family expectations are unrealistic. Occasionally, I'm afraid, it's sheer nastiness. They want to get rid of the old person, or want to sell the house or get them away for their own reasons. So you have to find out what's going on.

'If it is just senescence, I try to keep them out of hospital, whatever the relatives say. I believe it's cruel to put them into the kinds of wards I would have to if they have enough insight left to rail against it. We are particularly keen to make sure all community care has been tried before anyone is hospitalised. We bring in voluntary help, visiting nurses, physiotherapists, chiropodists and so on. Or we try to get them into supervised accommodation. But local authorities have limited resources and it's a fight to get a place. And now that the over-75s are increasing in number, there will be even heavier demands.'

Tom Arie, on the subject of family care in *Dementia in the elderly: diagnosis and assessment*, refers to the 'Monday morning syndrome', as being well known to general practitioners, psychiatrists and geriatricians. 'An old lady, often doing quite well, if not perfectly well, is living on her own and her children come for their quarterly Sunday visit. They see she could well do with rather more care than she is having, but are unable or unwilling to provide it themselves. They telephone the general practitioner "first thing on Monday morning" to say that "something must be done".' Arie also mentions the 'Friday afternoon crisis', brought about by the fact that those concerned with the patient – whether relatives or professional attendants – are planning to go away for the weekend.

Very often, relatives will go to a doctor and say, 'She's got to go, you know. She needs looking after. What are you going to do about it?' What this really means is, '*I* am washing my hands of her. What are *you*, doctor, going to do?'

What many people do not realise – until it happens to them – is that institutions cannot provide personal care. They can only provide second-class care – in the sense that first-class care is being at home with the family, and being involved. Move an old person who is already confused away from people he knows to people who are total strangers; from a group of people who know something about his background and share his memories, to others who do not; from a family environment into an unfamiliar one – and the decline in morale is rapid. Once in a home or hospital where everything is regimented, and they have little say in their own personal life, they give up and feel they have been abandoned. They need to be kept in the community in areas which are familiar to them.

However good the care of the home or hospital – and of course this varies enormously – the result is still that of a dumping-ground. When you walk into a geriatric ward, or the sitting-room of a home, you are immediately conscious of from ten to fifty slumped figures. They are often sedated, and their eyes are incurious. They watch television without comment or movement. This limbo land before death can last five or ten years or more.

Dr John Agate also makes the point that it is best, from the elderly person's standpoint, to stay at home among familiar people and things. 'Attempting to look after a patient in his own home, in relays with kindly help from neighbours and nurses if this is practicable, is much better than moving him around the younger generation's various houses in rotation, though sharing the burden like this is the means by which some families manage the job successfully and preserve some of their own home life.'

Not all families are intent on getting their elderly relations to a home or hospital. There are, for instance, over 300,000 single men and women caring for an elderly relation. A great many are devoted, and indeed have to have a lot of persuasion from the doctor to allow a parent to go to hospital, even when the task of caring is obviously beyond their capabilities.

Nevertheless, problems do arise. Sometimes, due to old family quarrels, the responsibility of looking after a parent falls to one particular brother or sister, who in time becomes resentful about this. The prospect of having to carry on caring for a parent indefinitely, without any prospect of relief or thanks for the burden they are shouldering, is also hard. In a survey carried out by the National Council for the Single Woman and her Dependents in 1978, it was found that the most common problems of the carers were loneliness and exhaustion.

The behaviour of old people who are confused or demented is another serious problem. A study in 1978 by Manchester University's Department of Geriatric Medicine on the problems of carers of stroke patients found that problems of behaviour topped the list. Understandably, under these various strains, families can reach the end of their tolerance and the ensuing crisis can lead to an urgent request to 'Admit Granny, or else'.

SUPPORT SERVICES

One valuable idea in helping with these problems has been the establishment of relative support groups in different parts of the country, such as that run from Bristol's Southmead Hospital, and at the Maudsley Hospital in London. These provide practical help – giving relatives a respite from 24-hour caring – as well as being a place to go to exchange information and advice, and compare and talk over the problems of coping with difficult elderly relations. At Bristol, help with transport and sitting-in is offered, as well as expertise from other relevant professions.

In addition to these relative support groups, there are other supports, such as voluntary agencies. Age Concern, for example, is a national organisation which acts as an information centre about the various services which are available for old people. Old people's welfare committees have been set up all over the country, affiliated to Age Concern headquarters in London, Edinburgh, Belfast and Cardiff. One of the aims is to correct the idea that old people are merely second-class citizens, and this is emphasised in its publication, *Manifesto: on the place of the retired and elderly in modern society.*

MIND (The National Association for Mental Health) is also concerned about the facilities, services and treatment available to the elderly. In 1978 it published *Mental Health for Elderly People*, a reply to the Department of Health and Social Security's Green Paper, *A Happier Old Age?*

Some of MIND's local associations run a number of projects for elderly people. These are intended to relieve loneliness and provide companionship and stimulation through activities for confused elderly people. Some are aimed specifically at providing relief for caring relations at home. They include the Park Club, run by the Buckinghamshire Association for Mental Health, which is a day centre for elderly confused people; a weekly social club for elderly people who have been mentally ill, or are at risk of being so (run by Enfield AMH); a day centre at Towcester for the elderly mentally ill (run by Northamptonshire AMH); and a day centre for confused elderly people, open twice a week (run by Sheffield AMH). A campaign officer, appointed by MIND and Age Concern, England, and based at the Sheffield AMH, focuses attention on the needs of the elderly mentally confused. Sheffield also started a scheme of home visits to elderly people who are unable to get to the centre. This is intended to provide relief for relatives. Southwark AMH has a similar 'granny-sitting' service. (Details of current projects can be obtained from MIND, along with the leaflet, *Who cares about Relatives*, which gives information on setting up relative support groups.)

Help the Aged, another national organisation concerned with problems of the aged, produces a newspaper called *Yours*. This contains a problem column called 'A Trouble Shared', aimed at helping the isolation and anxiety felt by the aged. And in a number of towns self-help groups for elderly people are now in operation, also aimed at ending widespread feelings of isolation and helplessness.

As well as getting practical advice from such organisations, families who are caring for elderly relations can also call on social workers to help with problems. However, as the MIND report on the mental health of the elderly points out: 'While social services departments talk of the increasing drain on their limited resources made by the elderly people in the community, the objectives of social services for this group generally remain unclear. There is a tendency to see the needs of elderly people being met in largely practical terms – by the provision of home help services, meals on wheels and so on.' (Home aids such as walking frames or commodes can also be applied for.)

A study carried out in Southampton in 1970 showed that most of the elderly clients were on a reserve list, and got intermittent visits by largely untrained social workers. Another in 1978, funded by the Department of Health and Social Security, also found that qualified social workers rarely took on elderly people, but that untrained social workers and social work assistants worked almost exclusively with them.

Although there is little coherent local authority policy in regard to mentally impaired elderly people, one or two initiatives have been tried out. In Avon, for example, the Social Services Department employed a group of untrained housewives who worked with elderly clients and reported back to senior social work staff. And Kent County Council pays members of the community on a contract basis to help elderly people – who have been assessed as being otherwise eligible for residential care – to remain in their own homes as long as possible.

A few local authorities organise holidays for the elderly mentally infirm. If relatives are badly in need of a break, it is also possible (if they live in the right area) to make arrangements for the elderly person to go into a geriatric or psychiatric ward for a couple of weeks; or even to a local residential home for an occasional evening. This is obviously unsettling for the person concerned, who may feel it is merely a prelude to a permanent place there. But it may be worth it to avoid a crisis. Health visitors also have a responsibility for working with the elderly, but there has been a growing trend for them to concentrate on families with young children. Community psychiatric nurses work with elderly people and in some areas, such as Buckinghamshire, they have been providing counselling and advice to elderly people and acting as a general link for other services.

Information on these services, and advice on accommodation, can be obtained from the social services department, health department, national organisations for the elderly, citizens' advice bureaux, and so on. Some elderly people suffering from dementia may be so dependent that the relative may qualify for a full or partial attendance allowance. Applications should be made to the social services department.

WARDEN-SUPERVISED ACCOMMODATION

This is appropriate for an elderly confused person who is liable to wander off or leave the gas on, but is still capable. Applications have to be made through the local council's housing department.

SHORT-TERM RESIDENTIAL CARE

Elderly people can be admitted, through their doctor, to hospital for short-term assessment, care and treatment. Or they may also be admitted to hospital or private homes for 'respite care' for the relations. In either event, if the elderly mentally infirm person is able to grasp what is happening, it is essential to explain the need for this short stay. Relatives, too, need to accept the situation. M. S. Batham, in *Home visits from a psychogeriatric unit*, says: 'It is often found that relatives fear or refuse to accept the patient home ... experience has shown that the best way to educate the relatives is to encourage them to visit the unit to observe the patients' reactions in hospital and study the way they are managed by nurses and occupational therapists ... the final stage involves the patient returning home on a day visit or trial leave.'

If more use were made of the short-term stay in geriatric hospital, for assessment and treatment of selected mentally infirm elderly people, psychiatric hospitals would not deteriorate into long-stay residences for unwanted elderly people.

LONG-TERM RESIDENTIAL CARE

By law, every local authority is obliged to provide residential accommodation for those who through advanced age or infirmity cannot manage alone. Some voluntary agencies also provide it. There are a few areas where local authorities have set up homes for the elderly mentally confused.

Social services departments are responsible for residential accommodation and hold lists of private residential homes. Conditions in both hospitals and private homes vary immensely throughout the country and some of the reports of the squalid conditions for elderly people in the back wards of Victorian mental hospitals, or in shoestring-run private homes, have been sad and upsetting. When you go into any geriatric ward or home it can be hard to come out without feeling depressed. Elderly people sit, sometimes comatose, in tears, or calling out for a nurse. There are too few nursing staff for individual attention, particularly with the constant demands of the elderly infirm.

The stigma of a psychiatric hospital remains – especially for elderly people, who consider the 'mental' hospital the end of the road. And lumping the 'elderly demented or confused' together in homes only worsens matters. The morale of both staff and inmates drops. Little can be done about dementia. But thousands of elderly people in hospitals or homes need not be there if our specialised services were used to support the front-line carers, such as relations, to cope with behaviour disturbance among elderly people.

9

Patients' Rights

Most patients in psychiatric hospitals and units are free to leave if they wish and only a very small minority are legally detained. However, there are occasions when this minority, or the friends or relations caring for them, are unsure of their legal rights. The following questions are those most frequently asked. The answers are in accordance with the Mental Health Act, 1959.

What are the different sections of the Act under which a patient can be compulsorily detained?

Under *section 136*, a person who seems to be suffering from a mental disorder in a public place may be detained by a police officer and taken to a 'place of safety' (usually a police station or hospital) for 72 hours. *Section 29*, also used in cases of emergency, authorises the detention of patients in hospital for 72 hours. *Section 25* authorises detention for a period of observation of 28 days. And *section 26* authorises compulsory admission to hospital for treatment for one year, with periods of renewal. Many psychiatrists go to great lengths to avoid admitting patients under a treatment order, and do so only after very careful consideration of the facts.

What safeguards are in force?

A person can be compulsorily admitted for 72 hours under section 29, in a case of 'urgent necessity' on the strength of *one* medical recommendation. A doctor – if possible the family doctor – has to examine the person. After this, he fills in and signs a form called a 'medical recommendation'. This form confirms that the person is suffering from mental disorder and needs to be admitted into hospital urgently and kept there for observation. One other form, called an 'application for admission', has to be filled in. This is usually done by an authorised social worker, but can be completed by any relation. It must be stated that the case is too urgent for admission for observation under section 25, which would mean a delay (because of the need, under section 25, to obtain a second medical opinion).

Section 29 is valid only for 72 hours. After that time, the person cannot be compulsorily detained and may leave the hospital, *unless*, within that time, a psychiatrist has examined him and co-signed a medical recommendation for further detention. If this happens, he is now placed under section 25 and no longer under section 29.

What safeguards are in force under section 25?

Section 25 allows compulsory admission into hospital for a period of observation of up to 28 days. This must be on the basis of an application by the nearest relative or by a mental welfare officer (such as an authorised social worker). The nearest relative must have seen the patient within fourteen days prior to the application. Two medical recommendations are also required. One of these should be signed by the family doctor, or a doctor who knows the person, and one by a doctor approved as having special experience in psychiatry. Both these must have seen the patient within seven days of each other and not more than fourteen days before signing the application. The application must also state that informal admission is inappropriate.

Once admitted under this section, as with section 29, there is no way the patient can extricate himself from hospital before the 28 days (or 72 hours in the case of section 29) is up (unless he is discharged) because the admission is meant to be just for assessment. Patients have no right to apply to a Mental Health Review Tribunal. But a patient formally admitted for observation cannot be detained for more than 28 days unless another application has been made for detention – which must not be just for further observation. The next step, if not release, is therefore an extension of stay under section 26.

What safeguards are in force under section 26?

Under section 26, a person may be compulsorily admitted to hospital for treatment for a period of one year. This can be renewed for one further year, and subsequent periods of two years, by the medical officer responsible. (This is defined as the doctor in charge of treatment.)

The admission procedure differs slightly from section 25. If a social worker makes the application, he or she must consult the nearest relative before signing it (unless this is totally impractical). If the relative objects – and informs the social worker or the local social services department of this – the patient cannot be put under this section. A social worker can, however, appeal to the county court to apply to overrule the relative. Two medical recommendations are required, just as with section 25, but a written statement by the two doctors as to the reasons is required.

Section 26 lasts up to a year. If the patient has not already been discharged by the end of that year, his responsible medical officer can review the position after examining him. If he renews the order, it will then last up to another year. If at the end of that year, the section is again renewed, it can then last for up to two years at a time before being renewed.

Under section 26, the nearest relative can order the patient's discharge. He or she must write to the area health authority stating the intention of discharging him, and giving the hospital seventy-two hours' notice. If the responsible medical officer considers the patient would, if discharged, be a danger to himself or others, he can stop the discharge by signing a report called a 'barring certificate'.

If this happens, the nearest relative can then apply to a Mental Health Tribunal for discharge. But this must be done within twenty-eight days of hearing of the barring certificate. After this certificate has been signed, the nearest relative cannot order the patient's discharge for another six months.

Also, if the patient is over sixteen, he can apply to a Mental Health Tribune to ask for his own discharge.

A couple of months might well elapse between applying to a Tribunal and having the case heard.

What are Mental Health Tribunals and how can they help?
They are independent bodies which were created to ensure that anyone

compulsorily admitted to hospital was not kept there unnecessarily. (The exception is those people admitted under section 65, which has a 'restriction order': in their case, the tribunals can only advise the Home Secretary.) Tribunals are organised on a regional basis. Each hearing is conducted by three members: a medical and a lay person and a lawyer (who is the chairman). The tribunal's only powers are to decide whether or not a patient can be released from hospital. It can compel witnesses to be present, and take evidence under oath. The hearings are usually held in private, in the hospital, although a public hearing may be requested. (There have, in fact, been only a few public hearings since the tribunals started in 1960.) The tribunal has the power to overrule the medical officer, if the patient is under section 26, and order his discharge.

To apply, the patient must ask the hospital for an application form and send it to his local tribunal (addresses below). His nearest relative can also apply on his behalf. Under section 26, the patient can apply: once within the first six months of admission; once during the second year of detention; once during every subsequent two-year period; within 28 days of being told he had been reclassified under another section.

London Office
16–19 Gresse Street
London W1P 1PB
North-East Yorkshire and
Midlands Office
Spur A, Block 5
Government Buildings
Chalfont Drive
Western Boulevard
Nottingham NG8 3RZ

North-West Office
St Martin's House
Stanley Precinct
Bootle
Liverpool L69 9BT
Welsh Office
Pearl Assurance House
Greyfriars Road
Cardiff CF1 3RT

Only about 12 per cent of those admitted under section 26 appeal to a tribunal (though regional figures vary widely). One reason is that those who are too sedated, hampered by their illness, or depressed, may feel too helpless to prepare their case; or else be unaware of their rights. Patients should be given a leaflet explaining these on their arrival at hospital. But if, during their stay there, they should need help over problems like a tribunal application, it is best for them to discuss these with a social worker.

MIND's legal department will always advise over any problems to do with the application, and will provide patients with trained representatives at a tribunal – usually free of charge. It always helps if a patient's case is presented by a solicitor, or even a friend or relative. MIND's leaflet *A Mental Health Review Tribunal May Help You* explains how and when to apply to a tribunal. This should be available through the hospital social worker, a community health council, a citizens' advice bureau or through MIND.

The tribunal psychiatrist will examine the patient just before or on the day of the hearing. The patient can speak at the hearing, and tell the tribunal why he thinks he should be discharged. Both the patient and the medical officer responsible can call and question witnesses. The tribunal's verdict is usually given within a week. Appeals to tribunals are not always successful. What is helpful, in getting a discharge, is for the patient to show he has somewhere to live, or someone to look after him, or has means outside the hospital. MIND has published a book by Larry Gostin and Elaine Rassaby, *Representing the Mentally Ill and Handicapped: a guide to mental health review tribunals*, which comprehensively explains how to prepare a case for a tribunal.

Who is my nearest relative?
In order, it is:

1	Husband or wife	6	Grandparent
2	Son or daughter	7	Grandchild
3	Father	8	Uncle or aunt
4	Mother	9	Nephew or niece
5	Brother or sister		

If the patient has been living with a member of the opposite sex as husband or wife for six months or more, this person will be counted as the nearest relative. But if there has been a permanent separation from either husband or wife, or one of these has deserted and not returned, then the husband or wife will not be counted as the nearest relative.

RECLASSIFICATION

Supposing the mental disorder the person is suffering from changes in some way, his medical officer, if he thinks this, can write to the area health authority to inform them. The patient is then reclassified. If this happens, he and his nearest relative must be informed. The patient then has the right to apply to a mental health tribunal within twenty-eight days to ask for a discharge.

As an informal or voluntary patient, what are my rights?
You have the right to leave the hospital whenever you choose, even against medical advice, and also to refuse treatment. However, it is possible in those circumstances that the psychiatrist in charge could change your standing from voluntary to compulsory – provided this is done in accordance with the conditions required for the particular section.

Can my status ever change from compulsorily detained to voluntary?
You can ask the psychiatrist in charge of your treatment if he would change your status to that of a voluntary patient. If your request is refused, you can then contact the hospital administrator and take your case to him.

As a compulsorily detained patient, can I ever take leave from the hospital?
As you improve, the doctor is likely to grant you permission to leave the hospital for various lengths of time. If this leave runs continuously for six months, you will be discharged. But if you leave the hospital yourself, without permission, you can be returned against your will by a staff member, social worker, or a policeman. If you are absent for twenty-eight days while under a section without a restriction order, your discharge is automatic unless you are classified as subnormal or having a psychopathic disorder. It is not illegal to go absent without leave from the hospital, but it is for someone to help you to do so, if you are compulsorily detained.

Can I vote while in hospital?
You can get your family to put you on the electoral register from your home address. If you are in a psychiatric hospital, the hospital

should put your name on the register (it doesn't matter if you are on twice, as long as you don't vote twice.) This is the situation if you are a voluntary patient. If you are in psychiatric hospital, under a section, however, you are not entitled to be registered on the electoral list, and therefore cannot vote.

Can I go on a jury?
Anyone who is resident in a psychiatric hospital, or is receiving regular treatment from a medical practitioner, is disqualified from serving on a jury.

What is the position on driving?
If you hold a licence, you must notify the licensing authority as soon as you realise you have any disability which affects your ability to drive. Consult your doctor if you are in any doubt about your capability. Notifying the authorities does not automatically mean your licence will be withdrawn, but it is obviously likely to be. Anyone undergoing treatment as an in-patient in hospital or nursing home is denied a licence to drive.

What about benefits?
After the patient's first eight weeks in hospital as a National Health Service patient, any sickness and invalidity benefit, widow's benefit, and retirement pension are subject to a reduction of two-fifths of the normal, full amount. The Department of Health and Social Security pays out amounts that are considered appropriate for personal expenses from time to time, if there are no other resources to pay these. *The Disability Rights Handbook* gives detailed information on benefits.

Are there any restrictions on mail?
Hospitals can open and withhold mail, under the Mental Health Act 1959, whether the patient is there voluntary or is compulsorily detained, if it is thought that it will cause distress or interfere with treatment. This is very unlikely indeed – though if it does happen the mail has to be returned to the sender as soon as possible.

Outgoing mail can be stopped if it is addressed to someone who has asked the hospital to stop the patient sending mail to him or her. It can also be stopped if the medical officer thinks it is unreasonably offensive to the addressee, or would be against the patient's interests in some way. However, the doctor may not open mail unless he considers the patient has the kind of mental disorder that may make him likely to send mail of this character.

Certain letters must never be withheld. They are any to:

1 The Secretary of State for Health and Social Security,
2 Any MP,
3 Any officer of the Court of Protection,
4 Your nearest relative, if you are under section 26,
5 The Mental Health Review Tribunal (as long as you have a right to apply for it),
6 A solicitor who is acting, or being asked to act, for you,
7 The European Commission of Human Rights.

What is the Court of Protection?

If the patient is considered incapable of making rational decisions and managing his own affairs – and owns a house or has savings or some other possessions of value – then the Court of Protection, which is in London, may appoint a 'receiver' to run the patient's affairs. This 'receiver' will probably be a relative, but can be a court official, and will do things such as invest any money, pay debts or carry out repairs. The patient's family might contact the Court of Protection and suggest a receiver be appointed. If the patient is against the idea, he can contest the case in court. He may require a lawyer or legal advice for this. MIND's legal department may be able to help here.

Can I get a second opinion?

If you are unhappy with the diagnosis or treatment you are receiving, you have the right to ask to be examined by an independent psychiatrist. You, or your nearest relative, must pay the bill.

Can I get a transfer to another hospital?

If you would like to be transferred to another hospital – because your family has moved, for instance – you must ask the hospital.

However, if you are not a voluntary patient, then you can be transferred against your wishes.

Can I get leave of absence as a voluntary patient?
If you are in hospital voluntarily, you can be given leave at any time. If you would like some leave, you must ask the doctor, or ward sister.

Have I the right to refuse treatment as a voluntary patient?
If you are in hospital voluntarily, you can refuse any kind of medical treatment – from tablets to surgery – and you should not be treated against your will. But refusing treatment may undermine your position: staff could threaten discharge or compulsory detention. It is best for you, or any relative involved, to try to discuss the problem with the staff concerned, especially if an alternative form of treatment available within that hospital is more acceptable. It may be necessary to contact the hospital managers to ensure your requests are adhered to. If, however, because of disagreement over treatment, the result is discharge against medical advice, this may well jeopardise your chance of readmission in the future. Help with a referral to another hospital or unit can be obtained through your own family doctor.

Have I the right to refuse treatment when compulsorily detained?
If you are compulsorily detained, the matter is more complicated. Some lawyers think it depends on what kind of treatment is proposed, and whether you are under a short-term or a long-term section. If you are being treated against your will, or it is proposed that you should be, you can contact MIND's legal department (22 Harley Street, London W1, telephone: 01–637 0741) for advice.

Can I be given electroconvulsive therapy (ECT)?
If ECT is prescribed, the doctor should ask you to sign a consent form. This will contain a phrase like 'the nature of which has been explained to me,' and it is important you do not sign the form until ECT has been explained, and you are sure you agree to it. The consent form is valid for a course of ECT, a certain number of sessions, and does not mean that you need go on having it indefinitely.

You can refuse the treatment at any time, even in the middle of a course, *despite having signed the consent form.* ECT can only be administered against your will if it is thought to be urgently necessary to save your life, or stop you harming others.

Although there is space on the form for your relatives to sign, giving their consent to your having ECT, as long as you are over sixteen, their signature does not affect your right to sign or not. The hospital may simply wish to have their signature too.

What do I do if I have a complaint?

If you have a complaint about any happening in the hospital, you can see the sector administrator informally, or else write a formal complaint.

If your complaint is about local facilities, you should contact the community health council for your district, as this is there to advise and help over questions about the Health Service, and can help with drafting letters and monitoring the outcome. The number will be in the local telephone directory under the list of hospital and health service numbers.

The community health councils, and any individual person, can refer a complaint about the inadequate working of services provided by the area or regional health authorities, or the family practitioner committee, to the Health Service Commissioner. He is appointed by Parliament and, like the community health councils, represents all of us as consumers of the Health Service. He cannot investigate the use of clinical judgement.

What should I do in an emergency?

Telephone your doctor or, if you are in contact with a social worker or community psychiatric nurse, telephone one of these. A few areas also have a crisis intervention team (sometimes based in a hospital, sometimes outside it) who take emergency calls. Most large district general and all teaching hospitals have a duty psychiatrist on call for emergencies (in other hospitals, he is not likely to be resident over-night). If you go to casualty with a letter from your doctor, it should be addressed to the duty psychiatrist, and not just to the casualty officer.

Can I get any financial help, outside hospital, with my standard medication prescriptions?
Check with your doctor. It may be possible for you either to get an exemption certificate, or else purchase a 'season ticket' for the pre-payment of prescription charges. A form can be obtained from the post office and this, after completion, should be sent to the local family practitioner committee. The card you receive in return must be shown to the chemist whenever a new prescription is required.

FURTHER INFORMATION

More detailed information on patient's rights can be found in Larry Gostin's *A Human Condition* (vols 1 and 2), published by MIND; *Patients' Rights Handbook* (also published by MIND); Gerry and Carol Stimson's *Health Rights Handbook* (published by Prism Press, Stable Court, Chalmington, Dorchester, Dorset); *The Disability Rights Handbook* (published by The Disability Alliance, 5 Netherhall Gardens, London NW3); *Notes to CHAR members on Liaison with Psychiatric Services* (published by the Campaign for the Homeless and Rootless, 27 John Adam Street, London WC2).

ORGANISATIONS

1   MIND (the National Association for Mental Health, 22 Harley Street, London W1 (01–637 0741). Leaflets available on patients' rights and advice can be obtained from its legal department. It will provide patients with trained representatives at a mental health tribunal. Its publication, *Mind Out*, gives information on treatment, mental health in general, local MIND associations, hospitals.
2   National Council for Civil Liberties, 186 King's Cross Road, London WC1 (01–278 4575). Gives advice on infringement of liberties.
3   Mental Patients' Union, 16 Clifton Gardens, St George's Road, Hull. Information group for patients' unions. Will advise on how to set these up.

EMPLOYMENT PROBLEMS AFTER PSYCHIATRIC TREATMENT

Those with any history of mental illness can find themselves in a very difficult situation when they try to get a job, even if they have been declared fit. As one young man in his twenties said: 'Having gone through finals, followed by nervous illness and spells in hospital and finally a good recovery, I find that when applying for posts this question of nervous illness always crops up in the forms to be filled in. The inevitable "regret" letter has turned up with sickening regularity. I sometimes wonder how much longer I can stand the jobless state without depression making me hopeless and apathetic.'

Others share the same feelings. 'I am now aged twenty-seven,' said one girl, 'and since nineteen I have suffered from depression, which necessitated various lengthy spells on psychiatric wards. I left teacher training without completing the course. I have now been declared fully recovered by my psychiatrist. When I apply for a job, how do I explain my lack of job experience? How do I write a letter of application; how do I fill in an application form? My own efforts have been fruitless. I did hold a clerical job for two weeks on a trial basis, but was dismissed. The reason given was lack of general clerical experience, but the general consensus was that someone had discovered my medical history.'

Employers are naturally concerned if would-be employees admit to having had psychiatric treatment or a stay in a psychiatric hospital, as serious problems can arise when employing ex-psychiatric patients. One man pointed out that, in his case, this was not so: 'My breakdown was a result of trials and tribulations, and I am not likely to suffer another.' The employer, however, may justifiably wonder whether a further breakdown will occur if the job proves stressful.

In one case where the employer overreacted strongly in this way, a woman was taken on as part-time secretary in a hospital, subject to satisfactory references. On her declaration of health form, she reported that she had received out-patient treatment for depression twenty-two years prior to her application. The offer of the post was withdrawn on health grounds: 'It is our opinion that the stresses and strain which pressures of the duties and sheer workload inherent in the post will impose on the occupant, make this an unsuitable appointment for you.' The woman had been in permanent employment for the preceding twenty-two years and had only had three and a half days' sickness during the previous two years.

Applicants are only too aware that disclosing any psychiatric problems may lose them the job. One teacher who had had a series of job applications fail said: 'I'm worried I will eventually have to accept some sort of factory or other routine job totally alien to my nature. Society still thinks that people who have had a breakdown, or some other form of mental illness, are then permanently unable to use their previous skills and abilities.'

If you do not wish to admit to a psychiatric history when completing an application form, this will naturally pose problems. As one secretary said: 'Some forms just ask general health questions, and they're OK. But others ask very detailed questions like, "Have you ever seen a psychiatrist?" or "Have you spent any time in hospital?" You'll never get the job if you answer truthfully, so you may as well not at all.' Her views were endorsed by others. A teacher, who had been under a psychiatrist for some time, and had also been in hospital with severe depression after a suicide attempt, said that he wouldn't dream of disclosing this in an application form. 'Well, I mean, who would?'

So what does one do? Simply disclose as much as necessary. Strike a balance between not appearing to cover things up and not over-stating the seriousness of the illness. Public employers seek medical references from doctors, so inevitably the details of treatment and condition come out. If you intend applying for a job, and you think your doctor may be contacted, it is sensible to have a talk with him in advance about this.

In one case, for example, where a girl applying for a job in Libya was turned down, she asked for an explanation and was referred to her doctor. He told her the company had requested information on her health and he had relayed the comments of a psychiatrist, made when she was on a psychiatric ward four years previously. She had been diagnosed as 'an acute schizophrenic'. 'It was just ridiculous,' said the girl. 'Ever since then, I've been working perfectly normally, sharing a flat, going on holidays abroad.' As she had hardly been to the doctor since, he was unaware of the extent of her recovery, and made no mention of this to the company concerned.

Undoubtedly, terms such as 'acute schizophrenic' frighten the layman, quite apart from causing the psychiatrists to argue over their precise definition. This can happen at an industrial tribunal. (Anyone who considers they have been dismissed unfairly – that is, due to their psychiatric history, rather than incompetence at their job – must appeal within three months to an industrial tribunal.) Ron Lacey, MIND's Social Work Adviser, points out that cases at industrial tribunals can get bogged down in a quagmire of psychiatric jargon. 'A GP, for instance, may jot down his thoughts – like, psychosis? manic? psychopath? – and the tribunal has difficulty in translating these into understandable behaviour terms. These working notes can later be seen as a firm diagnosis, when in fact the GP is really saying, "I do not understand what is happening here." '

In most cases, it is not possible to fire someone just because he has a history of psychiatric treatment. (Anyone who considers they have been discriminated against in this way should contact MIND's legal department for advice immediately.) However, information which has not been disclosed on a job application form may, if it is later discovered, invalidate the contract of employment. A psychiatric history may also be discovered when other problems arise involving lateness, sickness, behaviour, and so on.

Although MIND has a file of complaints from employees who have encountered a harsh attitude towards their past psychiatric history, many employers go to great lengths to help employees with psychiatric problems, allowing them, in some cases, generous time off to recover. But there are certain jobs in the public sector – for example, nurses, teachers, social workers – where there would be immediate newspaper headlines if there were any incident which called into question a person's past psychiatric history. In jobs like these, employers play safe.

Obviously an element of luck enters this whole area: two people can have quite different experiences with employers. MIND, meanwhile, is pressing for legislation similar to that contained in the

Rehabilitation of Offenders Act, which would make it possible legitimately to choose not to disclose a previous history of psychiatric treatment, after the elapse of a certain period of time.

APPENDIXES

APPENDIX I TREATMENT

There are a number of treatments for mental disorders. The main ones are as follows:

PSYCHOTHERAPY

This is sometimes known as 'talking treatment', as it allows the client to talk about his difficulties in an uncritical atmosphere.

Many people are consciously unaware of the reasons behind their disturbed state: by listening to them talking freely, the psychotherapist can help to interpret the factors that have caused this state. He can then suggest new and different ways of looking at the problems; can offer different interpretations of the way other people have behaved; and can help to change the person's attitudes and emotional reactions.

Sessions with a psychotherapist last half an hour or 50 minutes, as it is important that the client has time to express his feelings. The emphasis is on the client talking: the psychotherapist will refrain from breaking long silences, as the client may be wrestling over what he wants, or does not want, to admit.

Clients may feel that the psychotherapist is now responsible for solving their problems. But it is important that they make any decisions about their life themselves, or the psychotherapist will merely become a long-term crutch. The aim of the psychotherapist is to help the client to accept the circumstances of his life that he cannot change and to give him the confidence to alter any of these that it is possible to change. Deep emotions can be aroused in the client, who may transfer his intense feelings of like or dislike for another person to the psychotherapist – who, in the client's mind, becomes identified with loved or hated figures in his life.

Analytic therapy is the most common form of psychotherapy, but it requires serious commitment in terms of time and money. The therapist has undergone lengthy analysis, so has experience of being a patient.

GROUP THERAPY

Group therapy is a way of mutually exploring emotional problems, with the help of one or two group psychotherapists. The size of the group can vary, though it is usually between six and ten people. It will meet regularly, for about an hour or an hour and a half, over months or even a year or two. Members can get support and encouragement from each other, and the group serves as a means of releasing emotions like hostility or affection. Group therapy can be particularly helpful to those who have difficulty in making relationships or who feel isolated. It is the most generally available form of psychotherapy on the National Health Service. It can also be arranged through a private psychotherapist.

FAMILY THERAPY

Members of the family are seen together for a number of sessions, by one or more therapists. This takes place either in the home or in a clinic or out-patient department. It is now realised that family relationships are an important key to understanding many of the emotional or behaviour problems of one or more of its members. When patients are seen in the setting of their family, a therapist can often recognise the cause of a crisis more clearly. And family members are helped to say what they think and feel more openly – so that an emotionally charged family atmosphere can be understood and perhaps defused.

HYPNOTHERAPY

This form of therapy is frequently used to help people give up smoking or reduce weight; to help cure anxieties, fears, stammering, excessive blushing; and to create confidence. Many are nervous about hypnotherapy, fearing to be put in a trance, in stage hypnotist fashion. But there is no question of unconsciousness. When a person is in a hypnotic state, he or she is deeply relaxed, but quite aware of what is being said. In this state of relaxation, patients are open to therapeutic suggestions made by the hypnotherapist to help them overcome their particular problem. People are extremely suggestible when in a hypnotic state. The hypnotherapist might also use analysis to find out the reasons behind the symptoms; hypno-analysis can be used to take a patient back in time to uncover a repressed incident responsible for a present anxiety state. Anyone can set themselves up as a hypnotherapist without breaking the law: but, as with psychotherapy, ask a reputable organisation, such as the British Society of Medical and Dental Hypnosis, for a referral.

COUNSELLORS

Some counsellors specialise in certain areas – for example, bereavement counselling or marriage guidance counselling. Others offer more general support. They frequently act as sympathetic but uninvolved listeners, who can help a client accept the difficult but unchangeable circumstances he faces. They can help people to see other points of view and suggest practical ways of coping.

BEHAVIOUR THERAPY

Behaviour therapists believe that certain behaviour has been 'learnt' and can therefore be 'unlearnt'. Their techniques have met with particular success in the field of phobias and obsessions. (Treatment on the NHS is usually carried out by a hospital psychologist or therapist, after a doctor's referral.)

One of these techniques is *desensitisation*. The patient is relaxed – usually by standard muscular relaxation methods – and then over several sessions is shown the object he fears, or is taken into the situation he fears. Sometimes this is done in imagination alone, or through the use of pictures. The treatment is carried out in gradual stages until the patient conquers the fear.

With the *flooding* technique, which is carried out only with the patient's agreement, the patient is confronted with the phobic object, without escape, until he becomes used to it and his anxiety level drops.

With *modelling*, often used in conjunction with desensitisation, the therapist carries out a particularly feared action and the patient is encouraged to imitate it: for instance, with a cat phobic the therapist would hold or stroke a cat and the phobic would, in stages, practise the same action.

DRUGS AND THEIR SIDE-EFFECTS

Tranquillisers and antidepressants are aimed at changing a person's mood and emotional state. These drugs are not intended as a permanent cure for a patient's state of mind, but to help a patient over a particularly stressful time. As the side-effects of drugs, if not known or anticipated, can make a patient stop taking them, some of these are listed below.

Minor tranquillisers (like Valium, Librium) aimed at calming a person down, commonly induce drowsiness.

Major tranquillisers (like Largactil, Fentazin, Sparine, Stelazine) are more potent tranquillisers, widely used to reduce states of high anxiety, aggression and excitement. They are frequently used to maintain schizophrenics in a stable mood. Side-effects can include drowsiness, dry mouth, rashes, nose stuffiness, constipation, drop in blood pressure, blurred vision, weight increase.

Antidepressants are characteristically slow to work, sometimes taking up to two or three weeks to do so. They fall into two broad categories.

First, the *tricyclic antidepressants*. These are the most popular antidepressant medication and are used as 'first line' drugs in treating all types of depression, especially severe psychotic depression. Tricyclic antidepressants (like Tryptizol, Saroten, Domical) can have the following side-effects: drowsiness, palpitations, nausea, giddiness, unsteady gait, blurred vision.

Second, the *monamine oxidase inhibitor antidepressants*. These are prescribed if the patient does not respond to the above drug treatments, or if they are considered more suitable. They have a wide therapeutic range, usually being prescribed for patients with neurotic depression, anxiety states and phobic anxiety. Side-effects include: dry mouth, blurred vision, dizziness, headaches, muscle twitching, sweating, unsteadiness, constipation, nausea, vomiting, insomnia.

If the above two kinds of antidepressants are taken together, there is always a bad chemical reaction. The monamine oxidase inhibitor antidepressants should also never be taken with certain food and drink which contain the substance tyramine – for example, cheese, meat extract, broad beans, pickled herrings, yeast extract, chianti. Severe headaches and serious rises in blood pressure may occur as a result of such combinations.

Lithium carbonate is the main drug used for the treatment of recurrent attacks of mania, coupled with depression, and reduces the severity and frequency of these attacks (it is not known exactly why). Patients are permanently maintained on this drug and regular monitoring of the lithium level in the blood is required. It is important not to take an extra dose to make up for a missed one. Side-effects can include nausea, diarrhoea, fine tremor of hands, excessive thirst, passing excessive urine.

Many of the above drugs can be slow to act: the side-effects, however, can often be felt immediately. There is therefore a natural tendency to stop taking prescribed drugs before any beneficial effects occur.

ELECTROCONVULSIVE THERAPY (ECT)

Technique: the patient is relaxed, given an anaesthetic, and an electric current is briefly passed through the brain. It is not known why or how ECT works, but its effect on chronic, severe depressives can be dramatic. On some people, however, its immediate effect wears off and further treatment is necessary; on others, it has little or no effect. A course of ECT usually involves six treatments spread over two or three weeks. There is argument over whether it can cause memory loss. Patients must sign a consent form before this treatment is administered.

CRISIS CENTRES

The idea of crisis centres, or a crisis intervention service, is gaining ground in this country, although there are still relatively few. The aim is immediate intervention in a crisis by a team of specialised people – such as psychotherapists, doctors, social workers. The team – usually called in by a member of the family – will visit the family, and the person with the disorder, in order to provide active reassurance and support. Sometimes it is thought best to remove the person from the family for a short stay in the crisis centre itself, where again individual support is provided. The crisis centre is seen as an alternative to admission to a psychiatric hospital.

APPENDIX II   ADDRESSES

The following are addresses of some of the organisations which work in the fields covered in this book. The inclusion or exclusion of any name or organisation is not intended to imply approval or disapproval of their activities. These addresses are correct at the time of going to press.

Counselling and psychotherapy

British Association for Counselling
1a Little Church Street
Rugby, Warwickshire
(Rugby 78328)
No counselling on premises, but can recommend practitioners

Brook Advisory Centre
233 Tottenham Court Road
London W1 (01–580 2991)
Advice and practical help to young and unmarried on emotional and sexual problems, contraception (local branches)

Family Welfare Association
501 Kingsland Road
London E8 (01–254 6251)
Casework with families in difficulties or distress

Guildford Centre for Psychotherapy
3 Hillier Road, Guildford, Surrey
(Guildford 50455 4)
Counselling and individual and group psychotherapy

The Institute of Family Therapy
(London), Mary Ward House,
5 Tavistock Place, London WC1
(01–388 3872)

The Institute of Social Psychiatry
115/121 Newington Causeway
London SE1
(01–407 2311)
Treats people suffering from nervous and mental disorders in a social, as opposed to hospital, setting

Isis Centre, Darlington House
Little Clarendon Street, Oxford
(0865 56648)
Counselling and psychotherapy to those in emotional distress

Lesbian Line, London WC1
(01–837 8602)
Information, help and advice service

London Gay Switchboard
London WC1
(01–837 7324)
Counselling, advice service

London Centre for Psychotherapy
19 Fitzjohns Avenue, London NW3
(01–435 0873)
Individual, group and family therapy

Mental Health Advice Service
19 Handen Road, London SE12
(01–318 1330)
Crisis intervention, counselling

Paddington Centre for Psychotherapy
217–221 Harrow Road, London W2
(01–286 4800)
Individual, group, marital and family
psychotherapy

Rape Crisis Centre
PO Box 42, London N6
(01–340 6145, 24 hours)
Emotional support for those who have
been raped or sexually assaulted
(regional branches)

Stresses of Life Volunteer Enquiries
(SOLVE)
91 Wellesley Road, Croydon, Surrey
(01–681 6644)
Adolescent counselling

Tavistock Centre
120 Belsize Lane, London NW3
(01–435 7111)
NHS clinic providing individual and
group psychotherapy, family and
marital therapy. Referrals restricted
mainly to north London

Women's Therapy Centre
6 Manor Gardens, London N7
(01–263 6200)
Offers feminist psychotherapy to
women and their families. Individual
and group therapy and theme-centred
workshops

Schizophrenia

National Schizophrenic Fellowship
78–79 Victoria Road, Surbiton, Surrey
(01–390 3651)
Advice and support to sufferers and
relations. 130 local groups. Newsletter
and large number of publications and
leaflets

The Schizophrenic Association of
  Great Britain
Tyr Twr, Llanfair Hall, Caernarvon
Gwynedd, North Wales
(0248 670 379)
Information on latest treatments,
meetings, conferences, newsletter

Local associations of MIND

Anxiety and stress

Al-Anon Family Groups
61 Great Dover Street, London SE1
(01–403 0888)
Offers comfort, hope and friendship
to families of compulsive drinkers and
gives understanding to the alcoholic:
over 400 groups

Alcoholics Anonymous
P.O. Box 514, 11 Redcliffe Gardens
London SW10
(01–352 9779)
Helps to keep members sober and
other alcoholics achieve sobriety

Be Not Anxious
33 Broadview Avenue
Rainham, Kent
(Medway 34262)
Self help group

Institute for Behavioural Therapy
22 Queen Anne Street, London W1
(01-444 6030)
Private treatment for phobias and obsessions and stress management

Gamblers Anonymous
17/23 Blantyre Street, Cheyne Walk
London SW10
(01-352 3060)
24 hour service on 01-368 0316
Group therapy and practical help and advice. Partners and parents invited

Open Door Association
c/o 447 Pensby Road
Heswall, Merseyside
(051-648-2022)

Self-help organisation and information service for those who suffer anxiety/agoraphobia, to help alleviate the symptoms of same. Meetings, newsletter, supplies of books/cassettes

Phobics Society
4 Cheltenham Road, Manchester
(061-881-1937)
Relief and rehabilitation of sufferers from agoraphobia and other phobic conditions. Self-help groups throughout country. Advice given on how and where to obtain specialist treatment and on self-help. Newsletters

Relaxation for Living
29 Burwood Park Road
Walton on Thames, Surrey
(Walton on Thames 27826)
Information, advice, classes, leaflets, tapes

Depression

British Society of Medical and Dental
  Hypnotherapists
42 Links Road, Ashtead, Surrey

Compassionate Friends
50 Woodwaye, Watford, Hertfordshire
(92 24279)
Help and friendship from and to bereaved parents

CRUSE clubs
Cruse House, 126 Sheen Road
Richmond, Surrey
(01-940 4818)
Practical help and encouragement to widows, widowers and their children, to adapt

Depressives Anonymous
(Keith Middleton)
21 The Green, Chaddersley Corbett
Kidderminster, Worcestershire

Depressives Associated
(Mrs Janet Stevenson)
19 Merley Ways, Wimborne Minster
Dorset
(0202 883957)

Families Need Fathers
84 Ulleswater Road
Southgate, London N14
(01-886 9176)
Support and advice for divorced parents

Gingerbread
35 Wellington Street, London WC2
(01–240 0953)
Self-help organisation for one-parent
families

National Housewives Register
(Gill Vale), South Hill, Cross Lane
Chalfont St Peter, Buckinghamshire
(02407 3797)
Encourages formation of groups of
women who meet together to discuss
topics of non-domestic nature. About
900 or so groups in Britain

National Marriage Guidance Council
Herbert Gray College
Little Church Street, Rugby
(0788 73241)
See telephone directory (under
marriage guidance) for local branch.
Confidential counselling service for
those having difficulties or anxieties
in marriage or other personal relationships

Acupuncture Association
34 Alderney Street, London SW1
(01–834 3355)

Post-natal depression

Child Bereavement Parents Help
   Group
5 Farringdon Avenue
St Paul's Cray, Kent
Help group for bereaved parents

Compassionate Friends
25 Kingsdown Parade, Bristol
(Bristol 47316)
Self-help for bereaved parents, local
groups

People Against Loneliness
12 Spire Hollin, Peterlee
County Durham
(0385 64411)
Information and advice

Prisoners Wives and Families Society
14 Richmond Avenue, London N1
(01–278 3981)
Support and advice

Samaritans
17 Uxbridge Road, Slough
Berkshire
(Slough 32713)
See telephone directory for nearest
local branch. Counselling for the
depressed, despairing, suicidal; confidential telephone support

Shelter
London Housing Aid Centre
157 Waterloo Road, London SE1
(01–633 9877)

Link Up
31 High Street, Lower Easton, Bristol
(Bristol 550562)
Tape recorded magazine for the
disabled and lonely

Mama
26a Cumnor Hill, Oxford
Support group for women suffering
from post natal depression

The Masectomy Association
1 Colworth Road, Croydon, Surrey
(01–654 8643)
Non-medical service of information
and support to women who have had a
breast removed: includes volunteer
helpers who are ex-patients

National Association for the Childless
c/o Birmingham Settlement
318 Summer Lane, Birmingham
(021 359–2113)
Information, advice and support

National Childbirth Trust
9 Queensborough Terrace
London W2
(01–229 9319)
Preparation for childbirth and parent-hood. Informal post-natal gatherings for mother-to-mother support. 100 branches

National Coordinating Committee of
   Self-Help
Groups for Parents under Stress
29 Newmarket Way
Hornchurch, Essex
(Hornchurch 51538)
Coordinates activities of groups

National Council for the Divorced
   and Separated
13 High Street, Little Shelford
Cambridge
(02204 2544)
Promotes interests and welfare of divorced and separated: activities of clubs based on group entertainment

National Council for One Parent
   Families
255 Kentish Town Road
London NW5
(01–267 1361)
Runs social work service to help one-parent families: action includes letter writing, telephone calls, home visits, counselling

National Women's Aid Federation
57 Chalcot Road, London NW1
(01–586 0104/5192)
Support, advice and help to the mentally and physically battered women and their children. Nationwide network of temporary refuges. Over 100 affiliated groups

Parents Anonymous (London)
9 Manor Gardens, London N7
(01–263 8918)
Helpline for distressed parents. Nearly 50 groups in various parts of the country: information from above address. Helpline telephone numbers include: Leicester 886735
          Harlow, Essex 414444
          Swansea 460384

Still Birth Association
15a Christchurch Hill, London NW3
(01–794 4601)
Information, support and local groups

Tell-a-Friend
3 Crown Road, Milton Regis
Sittingbourne, Kent
(Sittingbourne 76746)
To help mothers of young children who are alone all day. Meets twice weekly; telephone service

U & I Club
9e Compton Road, London N1
(01–359 0403)
For sufferers of cystitis: advice and information

Anorexia

Anorexic Aid
12 Townsend Road, Chesham
Buckinghamshire

Mutual support organisation for anorexics and their families. Branches nationwide. Newsletter

The elderly mentally infirm

Age Concern
(National Old People's Welfare
   Council)
Bernard Sunley House
60 Pitcairn Road, Mitcham, Surrey
(01–640 5431)
Advice, information, publications and other services obtainable from over one thousand local groups

British Red Cross Society
9 Grosvenor Crescent, London SW1
(01–235 5454)
Clubs and day centres for elderly

Care and Counsel for the Elderly
10 Fleet Street, London EC4
(01–353 1892)
Advice on placing the elderly in London. Grants for nursing care for chronic invalids in need and help in raising money for other needs; general advice

Contact
15 Henrietta Street, London WC2
(01–240 0630)
Voluntary service providing companionship for elderly housebound people by introducing them to younger, more active people

Cruse
National Organisation for Widows
   and their Children
Cruse House, 126 Sheen Road
Richmond, Surrey
(01–940 4818/9047)
Provides counselling and advisory service and social activities

Easymind Home Care Service Agency
3 Oakshade Road, Oxshott, Surrey
(970–2087)
To provide care at home for the elderly (mainly)

Friends of the Elderly and
   Gentlefolk's Help
42 Ebury Street, London SW1
(01–730 8263)
Financial help where statutory help is not available; residential homes

GRACE
Leigh Corner, Leigh Hill Road
Cobham, Surrey
(Cobham 2928/5765)
Advice about permanent or temporary accommodation for elderly people, with or without nursing care. The service covers England, south of a line including Norfolk to Hereford and Worcester but excludes London

Help the Aged
32 Dover Street, London W1
(01–499 0972)
Fund raising charity for the aged in
need at home and abroad. Day centres,
national sheltered housing scheme.
Monthly newspaper, *Yours*

National Council for the Single
    Woman and Her Dependent
29 Chilworth Mews, London W2
(01–262 1451)
Provides information and guidance
for the single woman and dependent;
promotes holidays and other relief
services; supplies information about
nursing homes offering short-term
care for elderly and infirm persons.

SEMI
(Support the Elderly Mentally Infirm)
Westbury Park Methodist Church
North View, Henleaze, Bristol
(Bristol 312562)
Relatives' support group, lectures

Shaftesbury Society
Shaftesbury House
112 Regency Street, London SW1
(01–834 2656)
Clubs and holiday homes for the
elderly

Task Force
1 Thorpe Close, Cambridge Gardens
London W10
(01–960 5666)
Offers friendship and practical help
through volunteers; local branches

Patients' Rights

Citizens Rights Office
1 Macklin Street, London WC2
(01–405 4517)
Practical help and advice on welfare
rights

Court of Protection
Staffordshire House, 25 Store Street
London WC1
(01–636 6877, ext 203)
Protects and manages mental patients'
property

Disablement Resettlement Officer
(at local social security office)
Will help those with past psychiatric
illness to find employment

National Association of Citizens'
    Advice Bureaux

110 Drury Lane, London WC2
(01–836 9231)
Aims to alleviate personal distress and
confusion by providing free, impartial
and independent advice or information. Will approach other organisations
on behalf of an enquirer and act as
mediator. Nationwide

National Council for Civil Liberties
186 Kings Cross Road
London WC1
(01–278 4575)

Northern Ireland Association for
    Mental Health
Beacon House
84 University Street, Belfast
(Belfast 28474)
Counselling, advice, information

Patient's Association
11 Dartmouth Street, London SW1
(01–222 4922)
Deals with NHS complaints: gives
help and advice to individuals

Scottish Association for Mental
    Health
Ainslie House
11 St Colme Street, Edinburgh
(031–225 3062)

Protection of the Rights of Mental
    Patients (PROMPT)
c/o 2 Boxley House
Pembury Road, London E5
(01–986 9308)

Accommodation/Crisis Centres

Andover Crisis and Support Centre
17 New Street, Andover, Hampshire
(0264 66122)
Crisis intervention, emergency accommodation

Psychiatric Rehabilitation Association
21a Kingsland High Street
London E8
(01–254 9753)
Day centres, residential homes.
Referrals restricted to local areas

Arbours Association
41a Weston Park, London E8
(01–340 7646)
Provides short-term crisis accommodation and long-term supportive
accommodation

Richmond Fellowship
8 Addison Road, London W14
(01–603 6373)
Therapeutic communities of up to 20
people for the mentally ill

Mental After Care Association
Eagle House, 110 Jermyn Street
London SW1
(01–839 5953)
Provision for homes and hostels for
adults recovering from mental illness.
Referrals restricted to statutory
agencies. Nationwide

Simon Community (London)
129 Malden Road, London NW5
(01–485 6639)
Other communities in Belfast,
Glasgow, Liverpool and elsewhere.
Temporary and long term accommodation with counselling for ex-
psychiatric patients

National Association of Voluntary
    Hostels
33 Long Acre, London WC2
(01–836 0193)

General

MIND (National Association for
  Mental Health)
22 Harley Street, London W1
(01–637 0741)
Information and Advice Service

MIND's 150 or so local associations run group homes and hostels; social clubs; befriending schemes. Its branches have a casework and advisory service staffed by trained social workers. Their legal and welfare rights service will represent clients in court. Local facilities, self-help groups and psychotherapy services information also available, as well as wide range of publications on all aspects of mental health

Northern branch
486 Durham Road, Low Fell
Gateshead
(0632 871543)

Trent
Lawton Tonge Centre
8 Beech Hill Road
Broomhill, Sheffield
(0742 668800)

North West
51 Regent Street
Blackburn, Lancashire
(0254 663052)

Yorkshire
155 Woodhouse Lane, Leeds
(0532 453926)

Wales
7 St Mary Street, Cardiff
(0222 395123)

Scottish Association for Mental
  Health
Ainslie House
11 St Colme Street, Edinburgh
(031 225 4606)

Northern Ireland Association for
  Mental Health
Beacon House, University Street
Belfast
(0232 28474)

APPENDIX III   BIBLIOGRAPHY

John Agate, *Taking Care of Old People at Home* (Allen & Unwin, 1979)

Tom Arie, 'Dementia in the Elderly: diagnosis and assessment' (*British Medical Journal*, vol. 4, 1973)

Nicholas Bosanquet, *A Future for Old Age* (Temple Smith, 1978)

George W. Brown and Tirril Harris, *Social Origins of Depression* (Tavistock Publications, 1978)

A. W. Clare, *Psychiatry in Dissent* (Tavistock, 1976)

Vernon Coleman, *Stress Control* (Temple Smith, 1978)

Katharina Dalton, *Once a Month* (Fontana, 1978)

D. Russell Davis, 'Depression as adaptation to crisis' (*British Journal of Medical Psychology*, 1970)

Disability Rights Handbook (Disability Alliance, 1980)

Leon Epstein, 'Depression in the Elderly' (*Journal of Gerontology*, vol. 31, No. 3, 1976)

A. Goldfarb, 'Geriatric Psychiatry', in A. Freedman and H. I. Kaplan (eds), *Comprehensive Textbook of Psychiatry* (Williams and Wilkins, Baltimore, 1967)

Larry Gostin, *A Human Condition*, vols 1 and 2 (MIND, 1975, 1977)

Bernard Ineichen, *Mental Illness* (Longman, 1979)

D. A. W. Johnson, 'Treatment of Depression in General Practice' (*British Medical Journal*, vol. 2, 1973)

T. G. Judge, 'Drugs and Dementia', in W. F. Anderson and T. G. Judge (eds), *Geriatric Medicine* (Academic Press, 1974)

R. S. Kalucy, A. H. Crisp, J. H. Lacey and Britta Harding, 'Prevalence and Prognosis in Anorexia Nervosa' (*Australian and New Zealand Journal of Psychiatry*, 1977)

Kenneth M. G. Keddie, *Action with the Elderly* (Pergamon Press, 1978)

Sheila Kitzinger, *Some Mothers' Experiences of Induced Labour* (National Childbirth Trust, 1975 and 1978)

Living with Schizophrenia – by the Relatives (National Schizophrenic Fellowship)

J. Wallace McCulloch and Herschel A. Prins, *Signs of Stress* (Woburn Press, 1978)

Richard Mackarness, *Not All in the Mind* (Pan, 1976)

Christopher Macy and Frank Falkner, *Pregnancy and Birth* (Harper & Row, 1979)

Isaac Marks, *Living with Fear* (McGraw Hill, 1979)

Ian A. C. Martin, *The Art and Practice of Relaxation* (Hodder & Stoughton, 1977)

Molly Meacher (ed.), *New Methods of Mental Health Care* (Pergamon Press, 1979)

Medical, Social and Psychological Aspects of Stroke (Report by the Department of Geriatric Medicine, University of Manchester, 1978)

Mental Health of Elderly People (MIND, 1979)

Angela Phillips and Jill Rakusen, *Our Bodies Ourselves* (Penguin, 1978)

'Psychotropic Drugs in General Practice' (Report on symposium, *British Clinical Journal*, August 1973)

Allen Raskin and Lissy F. Jarvik, *Psychiatric Symptoms and Cognitive Loss in the Elderly* (John Wiley, 1979)

Leon Salzman, *The Obsessive Personality* (New York, Jason Aronson, 1973)

Schizophrenia? (Office of Health Economics)

Services for Mental Illness Related to Old Age (HMSO, 1972)

David Stafford-Clark and Andrew C. Smith, *Psychiatry for Students* (Allen & Unwin, 1978)

Charles Spielberger, *Understanding Stress and Anxiety* (Harper & Row, 1979)

Gerry and Carol Stimson, *Health Rights Handbook* (Prism Press, 1978)

Stuart Sutherland, *Breakdown* (Granada Publishing, 1977)

Alexandra Symonds, 'Phobias after marriage: women's declaration of dependence', in Jean Baker Miller (ed.), *Psychoanalysis and Women* (Penguin, 1973)

Peter Townsend and D. Wedderburn, *The Aged in the Welfare State* (G. Bell, 1962)

Eileen Vaughan, 'Counselling Anorexia' (*Marriage Guidance Journal*, September 1979)

J. K. Wing and Clare Creer, *Schizophrenia at Home* (National Schizophrenic Fellowship, 1974)